Dad's Guide to VBAC: Navigating the Journey of Vaginal Birth After Cesarean

Chad Patterson

If you are picking up this book, there is a good chance you have a wife or birthing partner that is contemplating to attempt a vaginal birth after a previous cesarean. I am not sure how you feel about it, but something tells me that you are not on board with it or maybe just really scared as to what the outcome will be if attempted. Likely that is why you are here reading this book. Well let me assure you that you're not alone. Many partners have heard their wife's or partners' desires, and thought, "What in the hell are they thinking?"

In this short book, we will be looking at what a VBAC is. Is it safe? Is it dangerous? Why is it important to her? Am I good partner if I object? Am I a good partner if I let her do something this crazy? What are the chances of an issue when having a VBAC. How do you side with your wife against the advice of many doctors? What if we try and fail? And lastly but very important how do I understand what my wife is feeling.

This book is not a long read, but one that I believe is important if your partner is contemplating a VBAC. While I will offer you statistics, and examples this book is about coming to an educated assessment as to whether you can get behind your partner on this journey.

So along with Stats, science etc. I will also bring you along on my journey as a VBAC dad. Yes I have been there; multiple times. My wife has had 3 VBACs after 3

Cesareans. I will take you on my journey as I went from non-supportive to I guess we can try it, to being her biggest champion. In the end the decision on how you feel about it is up to you. I just ask that you read this and take in all the aspects around her desire before you make that decision, because as we will see this rabbit hole goes so much deeper and spreads out far wider than we could ever imagine from looking at it on the outside. If you want to understand just how deep and far it goes you have to get in and find out. Regardless of how you feel about it at the end, this knowledge will be vital no matter the outcome. If I had read what you are about to read, it could have saved years of emotional pain and need to heal for both my wife and myself. Now let's climb in and see just how deep and wide this rabbit hole goes.

We will look at why your wife or partner desires a VBAC on a deeper level in the next chapter, but know now that there are many reasons behind her desire. They are both physical and emotional. As partners; especially partners without a uterus, we tend to look at the birth from the physical aspects, but birth is much deeper and far more intimate than we could ever imagine. As you read this book, and discuss this with your partner you must open your mind to understand the birth process from both the physical and emotional aspects.

Chapter 1

What is a VBAC?

If you're reading this you may have been through this rodeo before with your partner, or it could be that you're being introduced to VBAC for the first time.   As mentioned in the introduction VBAC stands for Vaginal Birth After Cesarean.   If this is a new term for you, don't worry as it is new to many people.   So if VBAC is not only possible but extremely likely to be accomplished without complication, why have you not heard of it until now?

That is because, for decades, it has been said once a cesarean, always a cesarean. While far from being true, it is one of those misconceptions that sounds correct and is just accepted.   The problem is that when you do the research even just at a high level you will see that VBAC is very achievable.   In the last decade, the CDC has seen a steady increase in the VBAC rate and currently, they are seeking to see this rate increase by 3 to 4% per year over the next ten years at the time of this writing.   There are many reasons for this and we will mention them in more detail later in the book.   For now however just know that even though this term may be new to you, it is not some obscure, longshot pipe dream.   Rather it is an achievable reality that is growing by the year.

Just what is a VBAC? The term VBAC stands for Vaginal Birth After Cesarean. While the name in and of itself appears to be self-explanatory and simple, it can be much more than that. For some, it is easier physical healing after the birth. For others, it is emotional healing, while to others it will free them of the guilt they have given themselves, and for many, it might be a combination of all three. To us, it might be a simple medical term or decision, but to our wives or partners, it might be the biggest hurdle to emotional well-being that exists in their life. Whatever your take on her having a VBAC is, don't just look at the physical aspects of it. For her, it goes deeper, much deeper.

Let's start off by stating that if your wife has used the term VBAC, or expressed a desire to look into it, even if it came in the form of a passing conversation, I can assure you she has thought far more about and likely researched way deeper than that passing conversation would lead you to believe.

While it may sound crazy or even dangerous to think about a natural birth after having a cesarean birth, it isn't. So if it is safe, why is it not used more often? Well, there are many reasons why. One of which started at the turn of the century when the typical Midwifery model of care was replaced by institutionalized care by OBs and Drs. Though midwives are still not as prominent as they once were, there has been a resurgence in recent years, as well as OBs opting to include more natural-minded birth practices in their model of care for their patients. Studies throughout the years, have led organizations like ACOG, the CDC, and WHO, to start pushing to reduce the number of Cesarean births and increase the number of natural and VBAC births.

Let me be very clear this book is not intended in any way shape, form, or fashion to be anti-cesarean. We intend to state that cesareans should not normally be the first approach and should be avoided if they can be. Cesareans do have their place, and they along with the medical teams performing them have saved countless lives of mothers and infants. When needed they are a godsend and we are lucky to live in a time when such options are available.

When is one needed? Well, there are numerous medical reasons why they are needed, and maybe even a personal reason a mother wants one. Again this book was not written to dissuade you away from a cesarean, but to simply show that there are other options, ultimately it is a decision that is between your wife or partner and their provider, but your support is always something they need as well. In the next chapter, we will attempt to try and give you a glimpse into what is going through her mind.

Chapter 2 Why she is mourning her healthy baby

This chapter is not meant to lay out the evidence or the pros and cons, but simply a chapter on how you can best support your partner's postpartum emotions whether it was her first Cesarean or her fifth. Not all women who have cesareans are going to have emotional trauma, but at the same time, not every woman who has emotional trauma will come out and say it. If she was wanting a spontaneous vaginal birth and wound up with a cesarean, there's a great chance she will be having some negative emotions about it. Now to be clear I am calling them negative emotions because they likely are negatively impacting her. Though they are negative, they are normal, and she should not be chastised, or made to feel like a bad person for having them. You can be there, listen, and ask how you can support her, but please do not attempt to tell her that her reaction is wrong.

She is mourning the birth she did not get, and everyone will mourn this differently. As long as she is not causing real harm to herself, or her other children, and yes even to you, just walk with her and let her mourn. She may need a little time to grieve and heal similarly as though a dear loved one was just lost. Support her but don't deny her a time to grieve. She may heal with a little time, but it might even require some professional help.

I know you love your partner and want to help her, but honestly, as hard as it may be to hear, you might just be part of her birth trauma, and even harder she may not even know that you are part of her trauma. A good gauge to answer this is how supportive of her having a VBAC, or avoiding a cesarean were you. If you found yourself on the side of the doctors and others suggesting a cesarean then you likely could be part of that trauma. Just like she is not a bad person for having traumatic emotions, you are not a ba person for suggesting or being neutral during the case for a cesarean. Likely you acted in the manner you did because you love your partner and you wanted what you thought was best for her and the baby, not because you were just ready to get it over with and move on. I remember standing in the room with my wife weeping as she was being prepped for her third cesarean. I thought it was the wisest decision, but at the same time, my heart was broken seeing her in emotional anguish.

I now know that she most definitely could have birthed vaginally and that the baby was perfectly healthy. Hindsight, education, and the eventual three VBACS allow me to see that now. At that moment, however, I genuinely thought it was the best thing for both her and the baby. It was not until later that I realized just how many emotions, dreams, and desires were being crushed at the moment, nor did I realize how viable and achievable a safe VBAC was. Though my love and care for my wife was no less than ever, in that moment she lay there alone in the world, her voice silenced. Though I stood beside her she stood alone.

Our daughter was born without issue, though not with the IGR the doctors were sure of and were basing the cesarean on. In the end, my wife lay there all smiles enjoying her new daughter while she was being sewn up. In my mind, all was well. Of course, I knew she was an emotional wreck before. That was obvious by the screaming at the nurse who we still to this day call Dragon Lady, as she was in my wife's face and sounded like she had just downed a carton of Pal-Mal non-filters, and was rude and harsh. My thought was once the baby is born and she is holding a healthy baby this experience will be a thing of the past. In the moments of immediate postpartum, I seemed right. Other than us joking about Dragon Lady, all conversations were joyous around our new daughter. Little did I know the tension and bitterness that were growing underneath the surface. You see I just THOUGHT that my assessment in the OR that day was correct. I had though made one grave error; I had divorced the idea of having a healthy baby from the emotions and grief of her birth. In my mind, since she was clearly in an ecstatic state of joy with our daughter, she was fine. For the most part, she thought she was too.

It wasn't until some time later that it all came out. I don't remember the length of time, but it was past the year postpartum before it all came to a head. She had noticeably been distant and withdrawn. While there was sex, it was almost like it was a chore for her. Several times I would ask, "Hey is everything ok?", and her reply was always that I was reading into something that wasn't there, and even in her mind this was likely the case. It was not until one night we were talking and again I asked what was wrong, only this time I kept asking and telling her that something was wrong, asking what have I done. All met with, "There's nothing wrong, and you have not done anything." Then it all came out. When she needed me the most I was not there. When she needed me to believe in her the most I didn't. Needless to say, that was a long night of talking, and for the good, I might add. I agreed that the next time I would hold firm with her until the end.

With this birth I had supported her VBAC attempt, even going out of state to speak with doctors. It was not until the very end that I stood in opposition. All the support during the pregnancy did little when I was not there in the moment that mattered most. So next time I would stand by her. Not just stand by her, but trust her, and believe in her. And that's what I did. I won't lie, I still had concerns, especially at the end. I had visions of losing them both or one of them to a ruptured uterus, but knew if she thought there was a need she would say so. This time we even had the doctor agree that if she could go into labor and show up to the hospital in labor she could have a trial of labor before a cesarean. We tried doing just that, and as we were getting dressed to head to the hospital, her water broke, and within 10 minutes I was holding our son in our living room. This time I had no choice but to support her, and it was what she says was her best birth yet, and the first of three VBACs after three cesareans.

Now neither of us recommend unattended VBAC attempts, as that was not our intention, but it was an amazing sight seeing her in her rocker nursing our son. She had a smile with all of our babies, but this one was different. This smile screamed I did it. She has accomplished a lot in life and now winning multiple awards in the birth profession, but that moment is still one of her biggest accomplishments. She faced the doubt of everyone, and proved that her body was not broken and that she could, and did prove their doubt wrong. To her in that moment she was like the athlete being told you're ot good enough for years, only to rejoice as she stood on the podium having the

Olympic gold medal placed around her neck.

That is our story, but yours will be different. I can't tell you what exactly she is

feeling, or who she blames, as I don't know you, her, or your situation. Chances are if

she is struggling after an undesired cesarean there is plenty of blame in her mind, you,

unsupporting friends and family, doctors, and even herself. Yes, she will probably be

blaming, and beating herself up worse than anyone.

So how do you help? Talk to her, listen to her, and allow her to grieve the birth

she lost.   Talk less, listen more. Your instincts may be like mine, and you want to fix

her. She is not broke, she does not need to be fixed, and she needs healing. Do not

minimize her grief. The number one thing I hear told to a grieving mother, is something

like, " This may not have been the birth you wanted, but you have a healthy baby, isn't

that what matters?" The one saying this is usually full of good intentions, thinking that

saying something along this line will help her see her blessing and she will realize that

she should forget about how the baby got here, and just be grateful they are here. It may

sound good to the messenger, but to her, It's a slap in her face. She hears "Your feelings

are bullshit, your grief is bullshit, you aren't grateful for your baby", and maybe more

depending on what she is going through. She can be fully grateful for her baby while

fully mourning the birth. Do not tie them together they are two separate things. Just

think about a time you lost someone dear to you, did you stop loving your friends and family because you mourned your loved one? No, and that is how she is with her birth and her baby. Grieving her birth does not detract from the love she has for her baby.

I said earlier, listen more than you talk. You may have to talk more at first, to get the conversations going. If your partner is like my wife she may be doing most of her suffering subconsciously, and not even realizing what is causing her emotions. Be gentle and probe slowly. Repeat this aloud I AM NOT TO TRY AND FIX HER, AS SHE IS NOT BROKEN. If you truly think she is grieving her birth ask her about it. Let her control the conversation.   If she begins to lay blame on you, resist your urge to go on the defensive, and trust me I know just how hard that can be. It's ok during the conversation to let her know why you did or didn't do what you did or didn't do but do so only so she can understand your choice, not to try and convince her you did the right thing. It's ok to say you just did not understand the level of desire she had, but ask her to explain to you why she wanted it so bad. Not so that you can counter, but so you can be equipped to stand by her better if there is a next time. Ask her if there is something you can read, or maybe a video you could watch to better see where she is coming from so you can better stand with her. She needs to know that you are doing this to be a better partner. If she gives you any material, read it or watch it. If you're not going to then don't ask.

As mentioned earlier, the fear of the unknown is not only a very scary thing but a very persuasive thing. Let her know that you want to go in armed with information next time. I knew my wife wanted a VBAC, and I knew she was researching while she was pregnant. She would tell me about this study and that statistic, but in reality, looking ack at what she was sharing with me versus what she knew was kind of like an iceberg. What she was sharing with me was the tip sticking out of the water, but what she knew was the entire iceberg. It's ok to say you did not know and ask her to help you understand. It will probably take multiple conversations, and may even need some professional counseling together.   Remember the goal is healing. She needs to be assured that you are in her corner and that you believe in her. Words can help greatly in the healing process, but it might not be completed until you are there in her corner as she births again. Would my wife have grieved her third cesarean regardless of my position? Yes she would have, but had I been unflappably in her corner until the end, it would have made all the difference in the world. It's one thing for doctors or nurses to not believe in her, but when her partner, the one that she trusts the most doesn't; well that is just a hard devastating blow.

Maybe she did have a cesarean, and there seem to be no signs of emotional distress whatsoever. That is great, as not all mothers will. If they had been anticipating or even requested a cesarean then their expectations were not crushed, thus less emotions around it. Just keep in mind that a cesarean may not even be traumatic until getting pregnant again. My wife had 2 cesareans, and emotionally there seemed to be no trauma. It was not until the next time she was pregnant that she began to show trauma from her previous one. Her first cesarean although somewhat dramatic left her with little trauma, as it was an emergency and was 100% necessary to save the life of our rainbow baby.

So do not just take for granted that there is no emotional trauma just because there are zero symptoms. It might be the next pregnancy if they surface, and leave you like, "Where the hell did that come from." If she has had a cesarean, don't be afraid to ask her how she feels about another one. It is possible that she would like to have a VBAC, but is afraid to share it due to fear of how others, including you, will respond. This could leave her dealing with this on her own, and leave you wondering what's wrong with her. Just giving her the channel to talk to you about it could mean the world to her. Desiring a VBAC can be an emotionally draining ordeal with support, but when she feels like she is going at it alone it can be crippling. Knowing you are there and in her corner could not only be the difference in her emotional well-being but also in her success with a VBAC.

If she is struggling after a Cesarean, assure her that her body is not broken, that she is not a second-class mother because she did not have a vaginal birth, and listen to her without trying to fix her or her situation, let her grieve. Do remember though that what she is feeling might be that she was abandoned in her time of need, or that no one believes in her. You may have been by her side every minute of the birth, but if she perceived she was alone, then that is all that matters in this situation. If this is where you find yourself currently then talk to her, listen to her, let her work through her grief in her time, and oh yeah listen some more. If need be, get counseling for her, for both of you and maybe even just you. If you do go for some counseling, then I would recommend using a licensed counselor who specializes in birth or reproductive issues. Do not just brush this off as her just being over dramatic. Work through it, and get help where

needed.

Chapter 3: Understanding VBAC

- *The history of cesarean sections and the rise of VBAC*

The history of cesarean sections (C-sections) and the subsequent rise of

Vaginal Birth After Cesarean (VBAC) reflect significant developments in

obstetric care, maternal health, and childbirth practices over the years.

Cesarean sections have been performed for centuries, although historically

they were often associated with high maternal and fetal mortality rates due

to limited understanding of infection control, anesthesia, and surgical

techniques. The term "cesarean" is believed to have originated from the

legend of Julius Caesar's birth, although historical records suggest that

similar procedures were performed in various cultures long before Caesar's

time.

Throughout much of history, cesarean sections were primarily performed as

a last resort to save the life of the mother or baby when vaginal delivery

was not possible or deemed too risky. In many cases, cesarean sections

were performed postmortem on women who had died during childbirth, as

attempts to save both the mother and baby were often futile without modern

medical interventions.

The development of anesthesia, antiseptic techniques, and surgical instruments in the 19th and 20th centuries revolutionized the safety and outcomes of cesarean sections. These advancements made the procedure more feasible and reduced the risks of complications, leading to a gradual increase in the rate of cesarean deliveries worldwide. With improved surgical techniques and medical care, cesarean sections became a more routine procedure for delivering babies, particularly in cases of fetal distress, breech presentation, or maternal health conditions that increased the risks of vaginal delivery. However, the rising rates of cesarean sections also raised concerns about overmedicalization of childbirth and the potential for unnecessary surgical interventions.

Emergence of VBAC:

In the late 20th century, as concerns grew about the increasing rates of cesarean deliveries and their associated risks, attention turned to the potential for vaginal birth after cesarean. The concept of VBAC gained traction as medical professionals and expectant mothers sought alternatives to repeat cesarean sections. The development of guidelines and protocols for VBAC, along with improvements in obstetric care and monitoring techniques, helped pave the way for its acceptance as a safe option for many women who had previously undergone cesarean delivery. Research studies provided evidence supporting the safety and feasibility of VBAC in selected cases, highlighting its potential benefits for both maternal and fetal health.

Challenges and Controversies:

Despite the advantages of VBAC, its widespread adoption has faced challenges and controversies. Concerns about the risks of uterine rupture during labor, particularly in cases of vertical uterine incisions or previous multiple cesarean deliveries, have led some healthcare providers to be cautious about recommending VBAC for all women. Changes in medical liability, hospital policies, and cultural attitudes towards childbirth have also influenced the availability and uptake of VBAC in different healthcare settings. In some cases, VBAC may be discouraged or unavailable due to institutional policies or provider preferences, leading to disparities in access to care for women seeking this option.

Current Trends and Future Directions:

In recent years, efforts have been made to promote shared decision-making between women and their healthcare providers regarding childbirth options, including VBAC. Guidelines from professional medical organizations emphasize individualized risk assessment and counseling to help women make informed choices based on their medical history, preferences, and values. The rise of initiatives promoting evidence-based maternity care, patient advocacy, and maternity care reform has contributed to increased awareness and support for VBAC as a viable option for many women. Ongoing research and clinical trials continue to explore ways to optimize outcomes and minimize risks associated with VBAC, with the goal of ensuring safe and accessible childbirth options for all women.

In conclusion, the history of cesarean sections and the emergence of VBAC reflect the evolving landscape of obstetric care and childbirth practices. While cesarean sections have played a crucial role in saving lives and improving maternal and fetal outcomes, the rise of VBAC represents a shift towards more personalized and woman-centered approaches to childbirth, with a focus on promoting safety, autonomy, and choice.

Benefits and risks of VBAC compared to repeat cesarean sections

Risk of Uterine Rupture: The most significant risk associated with VBAC is uterine rupture, where the scar from the previous cesarean tears open during labor. Uterine rupture can lead to serious maternal and fetal complications, including hemorrhage, fetal distress, and, in rare cases, neonatal death. The risk of uterine rupture is generally low but increases with factors such as a previous classical uterine incision, multiple prior cesarean deliveries, and the use of labor-inducing medications.

Failed Trial of Labor: Some women who attempt VBAC may experience labor complications that necessitate an emergency cesarean delivery. This can result in increased risks compared to planned repeat cesarean sections, including higher rates of maternal and neonatal morbidity.

Benefits of Repeat Cesarean Sections:

Predictable Birth Experience: Repeat cesarean sections are planned surgical procedures, allowing for a more predictable birth experience in terms of timing and delivery. This can provide a sense of control and certainty for some women and healthcare providers.

Reduced Risk of Uterine Rupture: Repeat cesarean sections eliminate the risk of uterine rupture associated with VBAC, particularly in cases where the risk factors for uterine rupture are elevated.

Risks of Repeat Cesarean Sections:

Increased Risk of Surgical Complications: Repeat cesarean sections carry inherent risks associated with abdominal surgery, such as infection, blood loss, injury to surrounding organs, and complications related to anesthesia.

Longer Recovery Time: Recovery from a repeat cesarean section may take longer compared to VBAC due to the surgical incision and associated discomfort. This can result in extended hospital stays, delayed return to normal activities, and increased reliance on pain medication.

Higher Risk of Placenta Accreta: Multiple cesarean deliveries increase the risk of placenta accreta, a potentially life-threatening condition where the placenta attaches too deeply into the uterine wall. Placenta accreta can lead to severe hemorrhage during delivery and may necessitate hysterectomy to control bleeding.

Both VBAC and repeat cesarean sections have their own set of benefits and risks, and the decision regarding the mode of delivery should be individualized based on factors such as the woman's medical history, obstetric considerations, personal preferences, and access to appropriate medical resources. Shared decision-making between the woman and her healthcare provider is essential to ensure informed choices that prioritize maternal and fetal safety while respecting the woman's autonomy and birth preferences.

Myths and misconceptions surrounding VBAC

Several myths and misconceptions surrounding Vaginal Birth After Cesarean (VBAC) persist, which can influence decision-making and contribute to misunderstandings about its safety and feasibility. Addressing these myths is essential for providing accurate information to women and healthcare providers considering VBAC. Here are some common myths and the corresponding realities:

Myth 1: VBAC is too risky.

Reality: While VBAC carries some risks, particularly the risk of uterine rupture, for many women, it can be a safe and reasonable option. Research has shown that the overall risk of uterine rupture during a VBAC attempt is relatively low, ranging from 0.2% to 1.5%, depending on various factors such as the type of uterine scar, number of prior cesarean deliveries, and use of labor-inducing medications. Additionally, careful patient selection, continuous monitoring during labor, and access to emergency obstetric care can help mitigate risks and ensure safer outcomes.

Myth 2: Once a cesarean, always a cesarean.

Reality: While some women may be advised against attempting VBAC due to specific medical factors or complications, many women with a history of cesarean delivery are eligible candidates for VBAC. The decision to attempt VBAC should be based on individualized risk assessment, considering factors such as the type of uterine incision, reason for the previous cesarean, maternal health status, and current pregnancy characteristics. For many women, VBAC is a viable and safe option for subsequent childbirth.

Myth 3: VBAC always leads to a uterine rupture.

Reality: While uterine rupture is a recognized risk of VBAC, it is not inevitable, and the majority of VBAC attempts are successful without complications. The risk of uterine rupture is influenced by various factors, including the type of uterine scar, number of prior cesarean deliveries, use of labor-inducing medications, and maternal age. Continuous monitoring during labor, adherence to labor management protocols, and timely access to emergency obstetric interventions can help detect and manage complications, reducing the risk of adverse outcomes.

Myth 4: VBAC is not safe for large babies.

Reality: The size of the baby alone is not a contraindication for VBAC. While fetal macrosomia (large birth weight) may pose challenges during labor, it does not necessarily preclude a successful VBAC attempt. Factors such as maternal pelvis size, fetal position, and progress of labor are more relevant determinants of vaginal delivery feasibility. Additionally, healthcare providers can employ various labor management strategies, such as patient positioning, fetal monitoring, and episiotomy, to facilitate vaginal delivery and reduce the risk of complications associated with large babies.

Myth 5: VBAC increases the risk of maternal and neonatal complications.

Reality: Research studies have demonstrated that, for many women, VBAC is associated with similar or lower rates of maternal and neonatal complications compared to repeat cesarean sections. Complications such as maternal hemorrhage, infection, and respiratory distress syndrome in newborns are not significantly increased with VBAC when appropriate patient selection and labor management protocols are followed. VBAC can offer benefits such as shorter recovery times, reduced risks of surgical complications, and improved maternal-infant bonding compared to repeat cesarean sections.

In conclusion, dispelling myths and misconceptions surrounding VBAC is essential for promoting informed decision-making and empowering women to make choices that align with their preferences and values. By providing accurate information, addressing concerns, and offering personalized care, healthcare providers can support women in making informed choices about childbirth options, including VBAC, while prioritizing maternal and fetal safety.

The importance of informed decision-making

Informed decision-making is crucial when considering Vaginal Birth After Cesarean (VBAC), as it involves weighing the potential benefits and risks to make choices that align with the individual needs, preferences, and values of the woman. The importance of informed decision-making with VBAC can be highlighted in several key aspects:

Understanding Risks and Benefits: Informed decision-making requires a comprehensive understanding of the risks and benefits associated with VBAC compared to repeat cesarean sections. Women need accurate information about the potential complications, such as uterine rupture and failed trial of labor, as well as the advantages, such as shorter recovery times and lower risks of surgical complications. Healthcare providers play a crucial role in educating women about the evidence-based information and guiding them through the decision-making process.

Personalized Risk Assessment: Each woman's eligibility for VBAC depends on various factors, including the type of uterine scar, reason for the previous cesarean, maternal health status, and current pregnancy characteristics. Informed decision-making involves conducting a personalized risk assessment to determine the suitability for VBAC based on individualized factors. Healthcare providers should engage in shared decision-making with women, considering their medical history, preferences, and values to make informed choices about childbirth options.

Exploring Alternatives and Preferences: Informed decision-making with VBAC also involves exploring alternative options and understanding the woman's preferences and priorities regarding childbirth. Some women may have strong preferences for either VBAC or repeat cesarean sections based on their previous birth experiences, cultural beliefs, or personal values. Healthcare providers should facilitate open discussions, address concerns, and provide support for women to make choices that align with their preferences and values. Access to Evidence-Based Information: Informed decision-making requires access to evidence-based information and resources to support women in understanding their childbirth options. Healthcare providers should provide clear and unbiased information about VBAC, including the risks, benefits, success rates, and potential complications, to empower women to make informed choices. Written materials, decision aids, and online resources can also supplement counseling sessions and support women in their decision-making process.

Respecting Autonomy and Empowering Women: Informed decision-making with VBAC respects the woman's autonomy and empowers her to actively participate in the decision-making process. Women should be encouraged to ask questions, seek clarification, and express their concerns or preferences regarding childbirth options. Healthcare providers should provide non-directive counseling, offer support, and respect the woman's right to make decisions that best suit her individual circumstances and values.

In conclusion, informed decision-making with VBAC is essential for promoting women's autonomy, ensuring personalized care, and optimizing maternal and fetal outcomes. By providing accurate information, conducting personalized risk assessments, exploring alternative options, and respecting women's preferences, healthcare providers can support women in making informed choices about childbirth options that align with their individual needs and values.

Choosing the right healthcare provider and birthing team

Choosing the right healthcare provider and birthing team for a VBAC (Vaginal Birth After Cesarean) requires careful consideration of several factors to ensure personalized, supportive care and optimize the chances of a successful vaginal birth. Here are some important considerations:

Experience with VBAC: Look for a healthcare provider and birthing team with experience and expertise in supporting VBAC attempts. Inquire about their VBAC success rates, approach to managing VBAC labors, and familiarity with the latest evidence-based practices and guidelines for VBAC.

Openness to VBAC: Choose a provider who is supportive of VBAC and respects your decision to attempt a vaginal birth after cesarean. It's essential to find a provider who values shared decision-making, respects your preferences and autonomy, and is willing to discuss the risks and benefits of VBAC in detail. Individualized Risk Assessment: Select a healthcare provider who conducts a thorough individualized risk assessment to determine your eligibility for VBAC based on factors such as the type of uterine scar, reason for the previous cesarean, maternal health status, and current pregnancy characteristics. Your provider should discuss the potential risks and benefits of VBAC specific to your situation.

Collaborative Care: Seek out a provider and birthing team who prioritize collaborative, patient-centered care and encourage active participation in decision-making. Look for a team that listens to your concerns, answers your questions, and involves you in developing a personalized birth plan that aligns with your preferences and values.

Access to Resources and Support: Choose a provider and birthing team who can offer comprehensive resources, education, and support throughout the VBAC journey. This may include access to childbirth education classes, lactation support, mental health services, and resources for managing potential challenges or complications during labor and delivery.

Hospital or Birth Setting: Consider the hospital or birth setting where you plan to give birth and ensure that it supports VBAC attempts. Inquire about the hospital's policies and protocols regarding VBAC, availability of labor support options such as doulas or midwives, and access to emergency obstetric care if needed.

Previous Patient Experiences: Seek recommendations and testimonials from other women who have attempted VBAC with the same healthcare provider and birthing team. Hearing about their experiences can provide valuable insights into the quality of care, support, and outcomes you can expect.

Ultimately, choosing the right healthcare provider and birthing team for a VBAC involves finding professionals who offer personalized, evidence-based care, prioritize your safety and well-being, and support your preferences and goals for childbirth. Take the time to research and interview potential providers, ask questions, and trust your instincts when making this important decision.

Assessing eligibility for VBAC

Assessing eligibility for Vaginal Birth After Cesarean (VBAC) involves evaluating various factors to determine the suitability and safety of attempting a vaginal delivery after a previous cesarean section. Here are some key considerations in assessing eligibility for VBAC:

Type of Uterine Incision: The type of uterine incision from the previous cesarean delivery is a crucial factor in determining VBAC eligibility. Low transverse uterine incisions are associated with lower risks of uterine rupture during VBAC compared to vertical or T-shaped incisions. Women with low transverse incisions generally have higher success rates and lower risks of complications during VBAC.

Number of Previous Cesarean Deliveries: Women with one prior cesarean delivery typically have higher success rates and lower risks of complications during VBAC compared to women with multiple previous cesarean deliveries. The number of previous cesarean deliveries may influence VBAC eligibility and success rates.

Reason for Previous Cesarean: The reason(s) for the previous cesarean delivery can affect VBAC eligibility. Some indications for cesarean delivery, such as breech presentation, fetal distress, or labor dystocia, may not necessarily impact VBAC eligibility if the circumstances have changed in the current pregnancy. However, certain factors, such as a previous uterine rupture or classical uterine incision, may increase the risks associated with VBAC and affect eligibility.

Interval Since Previous Cesarean: The interval between the previous cesarean delivery and the current pregnancy may influence VBAC eligibility. Longer intervals (e.g., $\geq$18-24 months) between cesarean deliveries are generally associated with higher VBAC success rates and lower risks of complications compared to shorter intervals.

Maternal Health Status: Consideration of the woman's overall health status, medical history, and obstetric risk factors is essential in assessing VBAC eligibility. Certain maternal health conditions, such as obesity, hypertension, diabetes, or placenta previa, may affect the safety of VBAC and require careful evaluation and management.

Current Pregnancy Characteristics: Factors such as gestational age, fetal size and position, presence of any pregnancy complications (e.g., placenta previa, gestational diabetes), and estimated fetal weight influence VBAC eligibility. Fetal well-being and maternal-fetal health considerations are important in determining the suitability for VBAC.

Patient Preferences and Values: Respect for patient autonomy and preferences is a fundamental aspect of VBAC eligibility assessment. Women should be provided with comprehensive information about the risks, benefits, and alternatives to VBAC and encouraged to actively participate in decision-making based on their individual preferences, values, and goals for childbirth.

Hospital Policies and Resources: Consideration of hospital policies, resources, and capabilities is important in assessing VBAC eligibility. Some hospitals may have specific protocols or requirements for offering VBAC, including availability of emergency obstetric care, anesthesia services, and surgical facilities in case of complications.

Assessing eligibility for VBAC requires a comprehensive, individualized approach that considers the woman's medical history, obstetric risk factors, preferences, and values. Healthcare providers should engage in shared decision-making with women, provide evidence-based counseling, and offer support throughout the VBAC journey to optimize maternal and fetal outcomes.

Understanding the factors that influence VBAC success

The success of Vaginal Birth After Cesarean (VBAC) can be influenced by various factors, including maternal characteristics, obstetric history, pregnancy characteristics, and labor management strategies. Understanding these factors is essential for predicting

VBAC success rates and optimizing outcomes. Here are some key factors that can influence VBAC success:

Type of Uterine Scar: The type of uterine scar from the previous cesarean delivery is a significant determinant of VBAC success. Women with a low transverse uterine incision typically have higher success rates and lower risks of uterine rupture during VBAC compared to women with vertical or T-shaped uterine incisions. Low transverse scars are associated with better uterine healing and lower rates of complications during labor.

Number of Previous Cesarean Deliveries: VBAC success rates may vary depending on the number of previous cesarean deliveries. Women with one prior cesarean delivery generally have higher success rates and lower risks of complications during VBAC compared to women with multiple previous cesarean deliveries. Multiple cesarean deliveries may be associated with increased risks of uterine rupture, uterine scar dehiscence, and other complications during labor.

Reason for Previous Cesarean: The reason(s) for the previous cesarean delivery can influence VBAC success rates. Women whose previous cesarean was performed for non-recurrent indications, such as breech presentation, fetal distress, or labor dystocia, may have higher VBAC success rates compared to women with recurrent indications, such as previous uterine rupture or placenta accreta.

Interval Since Previous Cesarean: The interval between the previous cesarean delivery and the current pregnancy may impact VBAC success rates. Longer intervals (e.g., ≥18-24 months) between cesarean deliveries are generally associated with higher VBAC success rates and lower risks of complications compared to shorter intervals. Longer intervals allow for better uterine healing and reduce the likelihood of uterine rupture during VBAC.

Maternal Age and Health Status: Maternal age and overall health status can influence VBAC success rates. Younger, healthier women with fewer comorbidities and obstetric risk factors tend to have higher VBAC success rates compared to older women or those with medical conditions such as obesity, hypertension, or diabetes. Optimizing maternal health before pregnancy and during prenatal care can help improve VBAC outcomes.

Pregnancy Characteristics: Factors such as gestational age, fetal size and position, and the presence of any pregnancy complications (e.g., placenta previa, gestational diabetes) can influence VBAC success rates. Favorable pregnancy characteristics, such as a vertex (head-down) fetal presentation and absence of obstetric complications, are associated with higher VBAC success rates.

Labor Management: The management of labor and delivery plays a crucial role in VBAC success. Continuous fetal monitoring, judicious use of labor-inducing medications (e.g., oxytocin), supportive labor practices (e.g., movement, hydration, pain management), and skilled obstetric care are important in optimizing VBAC outcomes. Healthcare providers should be prepared to manage potential complications, such as uterine rupture or fetal distress, promptly and effectively during labor.

Overall, VBAC success is influenced by a combination of maternal, obstetric, and labor-related factors. Healthcare providers should conduct individualized risk assessments, provide evidence-based counseling, and offer comprehensive support to women attempting VBAC to maximize the likelihood of a successful vaginal birth while ensuring maternal and fetal safety.

Creating a birth plan tailored to VBAC

Creating a birth plan tailored to Vaginal Birth After Cesarean (VBAC) involves outlining your preferences, priorities, and goals for childbirth while considering the unique aspects of attempting a vaginal birth after a previous cesarean delivery. Here are some key steps to create a VBAC-specific birth plan:

Educate Yourself: Start by educating yourself about VBAC, including the risks, benefits, and evidence-based practices associated with attempting a vaginal birth after cesarean. Research reputable sources of information, such as medical journals, professional guidelines, and organizations specializing in VBAC advocacy and support.

Discuss with Your Healthcare Provider: Schedule a consultation with your healthcare provider (obstetrician, midwife, or family physician) to discuss your desire for a VBAC and develop a personalized birth plan. Your provider can assess your eligibility for VBAC based on factors such as the type of uterine scar, reason for the previous cesarean, maternal health status, and current pregnancy characteristics.

Outline Your Preferences: Clearly outline your preferences and priorities for childbirth in your birth plan. Include details such as your preferred birth environment (e.g., hospital, birthing center, home birth), support persons (e.g., partner, doula), pain management options (e.g., natural techniques, epidural), and desired interventions or procedures during labor and delivery.

VBAC-Specific Considerations: Address VBAC-specific considerations in your birth plan, such as your preferences for monitoring during labor (e.g., intermittent auscultation vs. continuous electronic fetal monitoring), preferences for labor induction or augmentation, and your approach to managing potential complications or challenges during VBAC labor.

Labor Management Strategies: Discuss labor management strategies with your healthcare provider and include them in your birth plan. This may include strategies to support progress in labor (e.g., movement, position changes, hydrotherapy), methods to cope with labor pain (e.g., breathing techniques, massage, relaxation), and approaches to facilitate successful VBAC.

Emergency Preparedness: Outline your preferences and plans for managing potential emergencies or complications during VBAC labor. Discuss with your healthcare provider the signs and symptoms of uterine rupture or other complications, and include your preferences for emergency interventions, such as cesarean delivery, if necessary.

Communicate Your Birth Plan: Share your VBAC-specific birth plan with your healthcare provider, birth team, and support persons well in advance of your due date. Ensure that everyone involved in your care is aware of your preferences, understands your goals for childbirth, and is prepared to support you throughout the VBAC process.

Flexibility and Openness: Remain flexible and open-minded as you create your birth plan and approach childbirth. While it's essential to outline your preferences and goals, recognize that labor and delivery can be unpredictable, and plans may need to be adjusted based on changing circumstances or clinical considerations.

Review and Revise as Needed: Periodically review and revise your VBAC-specific birth plan as your pregnancy progresses and your preferences evolve. Stay informed about any updates or changes in your healthcare provider's recommendations or hospital policies related to VBAC, and adjust your birth plan accordingly.

By taking these steps to create a birth plan tailored to VBAC, you can communicate your preferences, empower yourself as an active participant in the childbirth process, and enhance your chances of achieving a safe and positive vaginal birth experience after cesarean.

Physical and emotional preparation for Vaginal Birth After Cesarean (VBAC) is essential to support a successful and positive childbirth experience. Here are some strategies for preparing both physically and emotionally for VBAC:

1. Educate Yourself: Gain knowledge about VBAC, including the risks, benefits, evidence-based practices, and factors that can influence VBAC success. Attend childbirth education classes, read reputable books and articles, and seek information from reliable sources such as healthcare providers, professional organizations, and support groups specializing in VBAC.

2. Establish a Supportive Care Team: Surround yourself with a supportive care team that includes healthcare providers (obstetrician, midwife, doula), supportive family members or friends, and other women who have experienced VBAC. Seek out providers who have experience and expertise in supporting VBAC attempts and who respect your preferences and goals for childbirth.

3. Address Emotional Concerns: Acknowledge and address any emotional concerns or fears you may have about attempting VBAC. Previous experiences with childbirth, cesarean delivery, or traumatic events may

influence your emotional well-being and confidence in attempting VBAC. Consider seeking counseling, therapy, or support from mental health professionals or support groups to process emotions and develop coping strategies.

4. Practice Relaxation Techniques: Learn and practice relaxation techniques, such as deep breathing, visualization, mindfulness, and progressive muscle relaxation, to manage stress, anxiety, and discomfort during pregnancy and labor. These techniques can help promote a sense of calmness, reduce tension, and enhance your ability to cope with labor pain and challenges during VBAC.

5. Stay Physically Active: Engage in regular physical activity throughout pregnancy to promote overall health, strength, and stamina for labor and childbirth. Choose safe and appropriate forms of exercise, such as walking, swimming, prenatal yoga, or low-impact aerobics, that help maintain cardiovascular fitness, muscle tone, and flexibility.

6. Eat a Balanced Diet: Maintain a well-balanced and nutritious diet during pregnancy to support optimal maternal and fetal health. Eat a variety of nutrient-rich foods, including fruits, vegetables, whole grains, lean proteins, and healthy fats, and stay hydrated by drinking plenty of water. Consult

with a healthcare provider or registered dietitian for personalized dietary recommendations and guidance.

7. Attend VBAC-Specific Classes: Consider attending childbirth education classes or workshops specifically tailored to VBAC. These classes may cover topics such as VBAC preparation, labor management strategies, comfort measures, coping techniques, and postpartum recovery after VBAC. Connecting with other women planning VBAC can provide valuable support and camaraderie.

8. Visualize a Positive Outcome: Practice positive visualization and affirmations to envision a successful and empowering VBAC experience. Imagine yourself progressing through labor smoothly, feeling confident and supported, and ultimately achieving a vaginal birth that meets your goals and preferences. Visualizing a positive outcome can help instill confidence, reduce anxiety, and promote a sense of empowerment during childbirth.

9. Communicate Openly: Maintain open and honest communication with your healthcare providers, birth team, and support persons throughout the VBAC process. Share your concerns, preferences, and goals for childbirth, and actively participate in decision-making discussions regarding your care. Clear and effective communication can foster trust, collaboration, and a supportive birthing environment.

By focusing on both physical and emotional preparation for VBAC, you can enhance your readiness for childbirth, cultivate a sense of empowerment and confidence, and optimize your chances of achieving a positive and fulfilling vaginal birth experience after cesarean.

Partner's role in supporting the VBAC journey

The partner's role in supporting the Vaginal Birth After Cesarean (VBAC) journey is crucial in providing emotional, physical, and practical support to the birthing person throughout the pregnancy, labor, and childbirth. Here are some ways partners can support the VBAC journey:

Educational Support: Take an active role in learning about VBAC, including the risks, benefits, and evidence-based practices associated with attempting a vaginal birth after cesarean. Attend childbirth education classes, read books and articles, and participate in discussions with healthcare providers to gain a comprehensive understanding of VBAC and its implications.

Emotional Support: Offer emotional support and reassurance to the birthing person as they navigate the VBAC journey. Listen attentively to their concerns, fears, and feelings about attempting VBAC, and provide empathy, encouragement, and validation. Validate their choices and decisions, and affirm their strength and resilience throughout the process.

Active Participation in Decision-Making: Engage in shared decision-making with the birthing person regarding their care and birth preferences. Participate in discussions with healthcare providers, ask questions, and advocate for the birthing person's preferences, values, and goals for childbirth. Respect their autonomy and support their choices, even if they differ from your own.

Physical Support during Pregnancy: Provide physical support to the birthing person during pregnancy by assisting with household tasks, preparing nutritious meals, and encouraging regular exercise and rest. Accompany them to prenatal appointments, ultrasound scans, and childbirth education classes, and actively participate in discussions with healthcare providers.

Assistance with Comfort Measures: Learn and practice comfort measures and coping techniques that can help alleviate discomfort and manage stress during pregnancy and labor. Offer massage, back rubs, or counter-pressure techniques during labor, provide encouragement and motivation, and assist with positioning and movement to facilitate comfort and progress in labor.

Advocacy during Labor and Birth: Serve as an advocate for the birthing person's preferences and wishes during labor and birth. Communicate with healthcare providers, convey the birthing person's desires and concerns, and ensure that their voice is heard and respected throughout the birthing process. Advocate for informed consent, shared decision-making, and respectful maternity care.

Continuous Presence and Support: Provide continuous presence and support to the birthing person during labor and childbirth. Stay by their side, offer encouragement, reassurance, and emotional support, and help create a calm,

supportive birthing environment. Be prepared to adapt to their needs and

preferences, provide comfort measures, and offer encouragement throughout the

intensity of labor.

Postpartum Support: Continue to offer support and assistance to the birthing

person during the postpartum period. Help with newborn care, household tasks,

and breastfeeding support, and provide emotional support as they recover from

childbirth and adjust to parenthood. Offer validation, encouragement, and

reassurance as they reflect on their VBAC experience.

By actively participating in the VBAC journey and providing compassionate, supportive

care, partners can play a vital role in promoting a positive and empowering childbirth

experience for the birthing person and contributing to optimal maternal and infant

outcomes.

Chapter 5: Navigating Pregnancy with VBAC in Mind

Prenatal care specific to VBAC

Prenatal care specific to Vaginal Birth After Cesarean (VBAC) focuses on optimizing maternal and fetal health, assessing VBAC eligibility, providing education and counseling, and supporting informed decision-making throughout the pregnancy. Here are key components of prenatal care tailored to VBAC:

Comprehensive Risk Assessment: Conduct a thorough assessment of the woman's medical history, obstetric risk factors, and previous cesarean delivery(s) to determine VBAC eligibility. Evaluate factors such as the type of uterine scar, reason for the previous cesarean, interval since the last cesarean, maternal health status, and current pregnancy characteristics.

Informed Consent and Shared Decision-Making: Engage in shared decision-making with the woman regarding her options for childbirth, including VBAC, repeat cesarean delivery, or alternative interventions. Provide comprehensive information about the risks, benefits, and alternatives to VBAC, and support the woman in making informed decisions that align with her preferences, values, and goals for childbirth.

VBAC-Specific Education: Offer tailored education and counseling sessions focused on VBAC, covering topics such as VBAC success rates, risks of uterine rupture and other complications, evidence-based practices for VBAC labor management, and strategies for optimizing VBAC outcomes. Address any misconceptions, fears, or concerns the woman may have about attempting VBAC.

Regular Prenatal Visits: Schedule regular prenatal visits to monitor the woman's health status, fetal growth and development, and progress of the pregnancy. Perform routine prenatal screenings, tests, and assessments to identify any potential complications or risk factors that may impact VBAC eligibility or management.

Nutritional Counseling: Provide guidance on maintaining a healthy and balanced diet during pregnancy to support optimal maternal and fetal health. Emphasize the importance of adequate nutrition, hydration, and weight management for VBAC preparation and overall well-being.

Physical Activity and Exercise: Encourage regular physical activity and exercise during pregnancy to promote cardiovascular fitness, muscle strength, and stamina for labor and childbirth. Recommend safe and appropriate forms of exercise, such as walking, swimming, prenatal yoga, or low-impact aerobics, and provide guidance on staying active while minimizing risks.

VBAC-Specific Monitoring and Surveillance: Monitor the progress of the pregnancy and assess for any signs or symptoms that may impact VBAC eligibility or management. Perform regular fetal assessments, including fetal growth ultrasounds and fetal well-being testing, to ensure optimal fetal health and readiness for VBAC.

Psychosocial Support: Offer psychosocial support and counseling to address any emotional concerns, fears, or anxieties the woman may have about attempting VBAC. Provide a supportive and nonjudgmental environment where the woman feels empowered to express her emotions, voice her concerns, and seek guidance from healthcare providers or support groups.

Preparation for Labor and Childbirth: Provide guidance and preparation for labor and childbirth, including VBAC-specific childbirth education classes, relaxation techniques, coping strategies for labor pain, and labor management options. Discuss the woman's preferences for labor support, pain management, and interventions during VBAC labor, and develop a personalized birth plan that reflects her wishes and goals for childbirth.

Continuity of Care and Communication: Ensure continuity of care and open communication between the woman, her healthcare providers, and other members of the healthcare team involved in her VBAC care. Maintain regular contact, address any questions or concerns promptly, and collaborate with the woman to navigate any challenges or decisions that may arise during the VBAC journey.

By providing comprehensive prenatal care specific to VBAC, healthcare providers can support women in making informed decisions, optimizing maternal and fetal outcomes, and promoting a positive and empowering childbirth experience.

Monitoring and managing risk factors during pregnancy

Monitoring and managing risk factors during pregnancy for Vaginal Birth After Cesarean

(VBAC) involves a proactive and individualized approach to assess and address potential

concerns that may impact VBAC eligibility or outcomes. Here are key steps for

monitoring and managing risk factors during pregnancy for VBAC:

Initial Assessment: Conduct a comprehensive assessment of the woman's medical

history, obstetric risk factors, and previous cesarean delivery(s) to determine

VBAC eligibility. Evaluate factors such as the type of uterine scar, reason for the

previous cesarean, interval since the last cesarean, maternal health status, and

current pregnancy characteristics.

Regular Prenatal Visits: Schedule regular prenatal visits to monitor the woman's

health status, fetal growth and development, and progress of the pregnancy.

Conduct routine prenatal screenings, tests, and assessments to identify any

potential risk factors or complications that may impact VBAC eligibility or

management.

Uterine Scar Assessment: Assess the integrity of the uterine scar from the previous

cesarean delivery through imaging studies, such as ultrasound or magnetic

resonance imaging (MRI). Evaluate the thickness and appearance of the uterine

scar to determine its suitability for VBAC and assess the risk of uterine rupture

during labor.

Maternal Health Monitoring: Monitor the woman's overall health status and

manage any pre-existing medical conditions or obstetric risk factors that may impact VBAC eligibility or outcomes. This may include managing conditions such as hypertension, diabetes, obesity, thyroid disorders, or other maternal health concerns through appropriate medical management, lifestyle modifications, and specialized care as needed.

Fetal Assessment: Perform regular fetal assessments, including fetal growth ultrasounds, fetal well-being testing (e.g., non-stress tests, biophysical profiles), and fetal movement monitoring, to ensure optimal fetal health and readiness for VBAC. Monitor fetal growth and development, assess for signs of fetal distress or anomalies, and address any concerns promptly.

Gestational Diabetes Screening: Screen for gestational diabetes mellitus (GDM) as per recommended guidelines to identify and manage any glucose intolerance during pregnancy. Gestational diabetes can increase the risk of macrosomia (large fetal size) and other complications that may impact VBAC outcomes, so timely diagnosis and management are essential.

Blood Pressure Monitoring: Monitor blood pressure regularly throughout pregnancy to detect and manage hypertension or preeclampsia, which can increase the risk of complications such as placental abruption or fetal distress during VBAC labor. Manage hypertension with appropriate medical interventions, lifestyle modifications, and close monitoring of maternal and fetal well-being.

Labor Induction/Augmentation Considerations: Assess the indications for labor induction or augmentation carefully and consider the potential impact on VBAC outcomes. Avoid elective induction of labor before 39 weeks of gestation to reduce the risk of uterine rupture, and use judicious use of oxytocin (Pitocin) for labor augmentation, if necessary, while closely monitoring uterine activity and fetal well-being.

Psychosocial Support: Address any psychosocial factors or stressors that may impact maternal health and well-being during pregnancy. Provide emotional support, counseling, and access to resources such as mental health services or support groups to help women cope with anxiety, fears, or emotional concerns related to attempting VBAC.

Shared Decision-Making: Engage in shared decision-making with the woman throughout pregnancy to discuss VBAC options, review risk factors, and develop a personalized care plan that aligns with her preferences, values, and goals for childbirth. Encourage open communication, informed consent, and collaborative decision-making to optimize VBAC outcomes and promote a positive childbirth experience.

By monitoring and managing risk factors during pregnancy for VBAC, healthcare providers can help identify and address potential concerns, optimize maternal and fetal health, and support women in achieving safe and successful vaginal birth experiences after cesarean.

Nutrition, exercise, and self-care during pregnancy

Nutrition, exercise, and self-care play crucial roles in promoting overall health and well-being during pregnancy, including for those planning Vaginal Birth After Cesarean (VBAC). Here are guidelines for nutrition, exercise, and self-care tailored to support a healthy pregnancy and optimize VBAC outcomes:

Nutrition:

Balanced Diet: Focus on consuming a well-balanced diet that includes a variety of nutrient-dense foods to support maternal health and fetal development. Aim for a diet rich in fruits, vegetables, whole grains, lean proteins, and healthy fats.

Adequate Hydration: Drink plenty of water throughout the day to stay hydrated, support circulation, and promote healthy amniotic fluid levels. Limit intake of sugary beverages and caffeinated drinks, and prioritize water as the primary source of hydration.

Prenatal Supplements: Take prenatal vitamins or supplements as recommended by your healthcare provider to ensure adequate intake of essential nutrients, such as folic acid, iron, calcium, and vitamin D, which are important for maternal and fetal health.

Healthy Snacking: Choose nutrient-rich snacks such as fresh fruits, nuts, yogurt, whole-grain crackers, or vegetable sticks to help manage hunger and maintain energy levels between meals. Avoid excessive intake of processed or sugary snacks that provide empty calories.

Mindful Eating: Practice mindful eating by paying attention to hunger and fullness cues, eating slowly, and savoring the flavors of your meals. Listen to your body's signals and respond to its needs for nourishment and satisfaction.

Exercise:

Regular Physical Activity: Engage in regular, moderate-intensity exercise throughout pregnancy to promote cardiovascular fitness, muscle strength, flexibility, and overall well-being. Aim for at least 150 minutes of moderate-intensity aerobic exercise per week, as recommended by healthcare providers.

Safe Exercise Choices: Choose safe and appropriate forms of exercise that are suitable for pregnancy, such as walking, swimming, prenatal yoga, stationary cycling, or low-impact aerobics. Avoid high-impact activities, contact sports, or exercises with a risk of falling or abdominal trauma.

Prenatal Exercise Classes: Consider participating in prenatal exercise classes or programs specifically designed for pregnant women, which offer guidance, support, and camaraderie with other expectant mothers. These classes may include exercises tailored to pregnancy, relaxation techniques, and education on pelvic floor health.

Listen to Your Body: Pay attention to your body's cues and adjust your exercise routine as needed to accommodate changes in energy levels, comfort, and physical capabilities during pregnancy. Avoid overexertion, excessive fatigue, or activities that cause discomfort or pain.

Pelvic Floor Exercises: Incorporate pelvic floor exercises (Kegels) into your daily routine to strengthen the pelvic floor muscles, improve bladder control, and support vaginal delivery. Perform Kegel exercises regularly, following proper technique and guidance from healthcare providers.

Self-Care:

Rest and Relaxation: Prioritize adequate rest and relaxation to support physical and emotional well-being during pregnancy. Get plenty of sleep, take breaks when needed, and practice relaxation techniques such as deep breathing, meditation, or prenatal massage to reduce stress and promote relaxation.

Emotional Support: Seek emotional support from your partner, family members, friends, or support groups to address any fears, concerns, or anxieties you may have about VBAC or pregnancy. Share your feelings openly, express your needs, and seek guidance from healthcare providers or mental health professionals as needed.

Mind-Body Practices: Explore mind-body practices such as mindfulness, meditation, guided imagery, or prenatal yoga to cultivate a sense of calmness, connection, and empowerment during pregnancy. These practices can help reduce stress, enhance self-awareness, and promote emotional resilience.

Bonding with Baby: Take time to bond with your baby during pregnancy through activities such as talking, singing, reading, or playing music. Connect with your baby's movements, respond to their cues, and cultivate a sense of closeness and anticipation as you prepare for childbirth and parenthood.

Self-Care Rituals: Incorporate self-care rituals into your daily routine to nurture your physical, emotional, and spiritual well-being. This may include activities such as taking warm baths, practicing gentle stretches, journaling, spending time in nature, or engaging in hobbies that bring you joy and relaxation.

y prioritizing nutrition, exercise, and self-care during pregnancy, women planning BAC can support their overall health and well-being, optimize VBAC outcomes, and repare for a positive and empowering childbirth experience. It's essential to consult with ealthcare providers before making any significant changes to your diet, exercise routine, r self-care practices during pregnancy.

Addressing fears and anxieties surrounding VBAC

ddressing fears and anxieties surrounding Vaginal Birth After Cesarean (VBAC) is an nportant aspect of preparing for a successful and empowering childbirth experience. ere are some strategies to help address fears and anxieties related to VBAC:

Educate Yourself: Knowledge is empowering. Learn as much as you can about VBAC, including the risks, benefits, evidence-based practices, and factors that can influence VBAC success. Seek information from reputable sources such as healthcare providers, professional organizations, childbirth education classes, and VBAC support groups.

Open Communication: Share your fears and anxieties about VBAC openly and honestly with your healthcare providers, partner, family members, or support persons. Expressing your concerns allows others to offer support, validation, and reassurance, and can help you feel understood and supported throughout the VBAC journey.

Address Misconceptions: Challenge any misconceptions or myths you may have heard about VBAC by seeking accurate information from reliable sources. Discuss your concerns with healthcare providers who can provide evidence-based guidance and address any misunderstandings or misinformation you may have encountered.

Positive Visualization: Practice positive visualization and affirmations to envision a successful and empowering VBAC experience. Imagine yourself progressing through labor smoothly, feeling confident and supported, and ultimately achieving a vaginal birth that meets your goals and preferences. Visualizing a positive outcome can help instill confidence, reduce anxiety, and promote a sense of empowerment during childbirth.

Seek Support: Surround yourself with a supportive network of family members, friends, or support groups who can offer encouragement, empathy, and understanding as you navigate your fears and anxieties about VBAC. Connect with other women who have experienced VBAC or are planning VBAC to share experiences, tips, and support.

Address Trauma or Previous Birth Experiences: If you have experienced trauma or negative birth experiences in the past, seek support from mental health professionals, therapists, or counselors who specialize in perinatal mental health. Processing and addressing past trauma or negative experiences can help alleviate fears and anxieties and promote healing and resilience.

Mindfulness and Relaxation Techniques: Practice mindfulness, relaxation techniques, and stress management strategies to reduce anxiety and promote emotional well-being during pregnancy and childbirth. Techniques such as deep breathing, progressive muscle relaxation, guided imagery, or mindfulness meditation can help calm the mind, relax the body, and cultivate a sense of inner peace and resilience.

Prepare a Supportive Birth Team: Choose healthcare providers and birth attendants who are supportive, empathetic, and respectful of your preferences and concerns regarding VBAC. Surround yourself with a birth team that listens to your needs, communicates effectively, and provides compassionate care throughout the VBAC process.

Develop Coping Strategies: Identify coping strategies and techniques that help you manage anxiety and stress during pregnancy and labor. This may include journaling, creative expression, spending time in nature, engaging in hobbies or activities you enjoy, or seeking professional support through counseling or therapy.

Focus on Self-Care: Prioritize self-care activities that nurture your physical, emotional, and spiritual well-being during pregnancy. Take time for relaxation, rest, and activities that bring you joy and fulfillment. Practice self-compassion, self-acceptance, and self-love as you navigate your fears and anxieties about VBAC.

Remember that it's normal to experience fears and anxieties about childbirth, especially if you've had previous challenging experiences. By acknowledging your concerns, seeking support, and actively addressing your fears, you can cultivate a sense of empowerment, confidence, and resilience as you prepare for VBAC.

Bonding with your partner and baby during pregnancy

Bonding with your partner and baby during pregnancy is a precious and important aspect of preparing for Vaginal Birth After Cesarean (VBAC). Here are some ways to strengthen your bond with your partner and baby throughout pregnancy:

1. Attend Prenatal Appointments Together: Whenever possible, involve your partner in prenatal appointments, ultrasounds, and check-ups with

healthcare providers. This allows your partner to stay informed about your pregnancy progress, hear the baby's heartbeat, and participate in discussions about VBAC preparation and childbirth.

2. Share Your Thoughts and Feelings: Openly communicate with your partner about your thoughts, feelings, and experiences during pregnancy. Share your excitement, fears, and hopes for VBAC, and encourage your partner to express their own emotions and concerns. Building open and honest communication strengthens your connection and fosters mutual support.

3. Create Special Moments Together: Dedicate time to enjoy special moments and create lasting memories as a couple during pregnancy. Plan date nights, romantic outings, or quiet evenings at home to connect, relax, and bond with each other. Take walks together, enjoy prenatal massages, or simply spend quality time cuddling and talking.

4. Participate in Childbirth Education Classes: Enroll in childbirth education classes together to learn about VBAC, labor and delivery, newborn care, and parenting skills. Attending classes as a couple allows you to bond over shared learning experiences, practice relaxation techniques, and prepare for the journey ahead as parents.

5. Practice Partner-Assisted Relaxation Techniques: Explore partner-assisted relaxation techniques such as massage, guided imagery, or breathing exercises to promote relaxation and reduce stress during pregnancy. Experiment with different relaxation techniques that help you and your partner feel calm, connected, and supported.

6. Read and Learn Together: Read books, articles, or blogs about pregnancy, childbirth, and parenting as a couple. Discuss your thoughts, questions, and insights from the readings, and explore different perspectives on childbirth and parenting. Sharing knowledge and learning together strengthens your bond and prepares you for the journey ahead.

7. Create a Birth Plan Together: Collaborate with your partner to create a birth plan that reflects your shared preferences, values, and goals for VBAC. Discuss your wishes for labor and delivery, pain management options, and support strategies, and make decisions together as a team. Your partner's involvement in the birth planning process enhances their sense of support and participation in the VBAC journey.

8. Practice Mindful Parenting: Embrace mindful parenting practices that promote present moment awareness, empathy, and connection with your baby. Spend time talking, singing, or playing music for your baby, and practice gentle belly-touching or visualization exercises to bond with your

baby in utero. Cultivate a sense of wonder and anticipation as you prepare to welcome your baby into the world.

9. Engage in Baby Preparations: Involve your partner in preparations for the baby's arrival, such as setting up the nursery, choosing baby names, and selecting baby gear. Collaborate on baby registry items, assemble furniture together, and take part in nesting activities that strengthen your bond and anticipation as expectant parents.

10. Express Gratitude and Affection: Take moments to express gratitude, appreciation, and affection for your partner's support and involvement in the VBAC journey. Show kindness, affectionate gestures, and words of encouragement to affirm your bond and strengthen your connection as partners and parents-to-be.

By actively bonding with your partner and baby during pregnancy, you create a foundation of love, support, and connection that enhances your journey towards VBAC and parenthood. Embrace these opportunities to strengthen your relationship, nurture your connection with your baby, and prepare for the transformative experience of childbirth and beyond.

Chapter 6: Labor and Delivery: The VBAC Experience

Signs of labor and when to go to the hospital

Recognizing the signs of labor and knowing when to go to the hospital for Vaginal Birth After Cesarean (VBAC) is essential for ensuring a smooth transition to active labor and timely arrival at the birthing facility. Here are some common signs of labor and guidelines for when to go to the hospital for VBAC:

1. Regular and Persistent Contractions: Contractions are the primary sign of labor. In VBAC, contractions may start as irregular and mild, but they typically become more regular, frequent, and intense over time. Time your contractions to determine their pattern and duration. When contractions are consistently strong, regular (usually every 5 minutes or less), and lasting about 60 seconds or more, it's typically a sign that labor is progressing, and it's time to consider heading to the hospital.

2. Increase in Intensity and Duration of Contractions: As labor progresses, contractions typically become more intense, longer-lasting, and closer together. You may notice a gradual increase in the intensity and duration of contractions over time. If you experience a significant increase in the strength and duration of contractions that are difficult to cope with, it may be a sign that active labor is underway, and you should prepare to go to the hospital.

. Water Breaking (Rupture of Membranes): The rupture of membranes, also known as the "water breaking," can occur spontaneously or as a result of medical intervention. If you experience a gush or trickle of fluid from the vagina, it may indicate that your amniotic sac has ruptured, and labor is imminent. Note the color, odor, and amount of amniotic fluid and contact your healthcare provider for guidance. In VBAC, the rupture of membranes may not always occur before labor starts, but if it does, it's a sign that labor is likely imminent.

4. Bloody Show: A "bloody show" refers to the passage of a small amount of blood-tinged mucus from the vagina, often accompanied by cervical dilation and effacement. It's a common sign that labor is approaching or underway. If you notice a bloody show, especially when accompanied by contractions or other signs of labor, it may indicate that your cervix is beginning to dilate and soften in preparation for childbirth.

5. Pelvic Pressure or Back Pain: Some women experience pelvic pressure, lower back pain, or a sensation of heaviness in the pelvic area as labor progresses and the baby descends into the birth canal. If you notice an increase in pelvic pressure or discomfort that is persistent and accompanied by other signs of labor, it may indicate that your body is preparing for childbirth.

When to Go to the Hospital for VBAC:

- Regular Contractions: When contractions are consistently strong, regular (usually every 5 minutes or less), and lasting about 60 seconds or more.

- Intense Pain: If you experience intense pain or discomfort that is difficult to manage at home.

- Rupture of Membranes: If your water breaks or you experience a gush or trickle of fluid from the vagina.

- Bleeding: If you experience heavy vaginal bleeding or other concerning vaginal discharge.

- Decreased Fetal Movement: If you notice a decrease in fetal movement or significant changes in your baby's activity patterns.

- Medical Concerns: If you have any medical concerns or complications that require immediate attention, such as signs of preterm labor, hypertension, or other pregnancy-related conditions.

If you're unsure whether it's time to go to the hospital, contact your healthcare provider or the labor and delivery unit for guidance. They can assess your symptoms, provide advice, and help you determine the best course of action based on your individual circumstances and VBAC history. It's better to err on the side of caution and seek medical evaluation if you have any concerns about the progression of labor or your well-being.

Coping mechanisms for labor pain

Coping with labor pain is a significant aspect of preparing for Vaginal Birth After Cesarean (VBAC). While every woman's experience with pain management during labor is unique, there are various coping mechanisms and techniques that can help manage discomfort and promote relaxation and comfort during VBAC labor. Here are some coping mechanisms for labor pain in VBAC:

Education and Preparation: Educate yourself about the labor process, pain management options, and coping techniques available for VBAC. Attend childbirth education classes, read books, and discuss pain management strategies with your healthcare provider to feel more informed and empowered during labor.

Breathing Techniques: Practice deep breathing exercises to promote relaxation and manage pain during contractions. Techniques such as slow breathing, rhythmic breathing, or patterned breathing can help distract from pain, increase oxygenation, and reduce tension in the body.

Visualization and Guided Imagery: Use visualization and guided imagery techniques to create mental images of relaxation, comfort, and progress during labor. Imagine yourself in a peaceful and serene environment, visualize your baby's descent through the birth canal, or focus on positive affirmations to promote feelings of empowerment and confidence.

Positioning and Movement: Experiment with different positions and movements to find what feels most comfortable and effective for managing labor pain. Change positions frequently, such as walking, swaying, rocking, squatting, or using a birthing ball, to help facilitate labor progress and alleviate discomfort.

Massage and Touch: Receive massage or gentle touch from your partner, doula, or support person to help ease tension, promote relaxation, and provide comfort during labor. Focus on areas of tension, such as the lower back, shoulders, or hips, and use gentle pressure or circular motions to soothe sore muscles and promote relaxation.

Heat and Cold Therapy: Apply heat or cold therapy to areas of discomfort during labor to help alleviate pain and provide relief. Use a warm compress, heating pad, or warm shower to relax tense muscles and increase blood flow. Alternatively, apply cold packs or ice packs to numb sore areas and reduce inflammation.

Hydrotherapy: Take advantage of hydrotherapy options, such as soaking in a warm bath or using a birthing pool, to help manage labor pain and promote relaxation. Buoyancy in water can relieve pressure on the body, reduce pain intensity, and provide a soothing environment for labor progress.

Music and Relaxation Techniques: Listen to calming music, nature sounds, or guided relaxation recordings to create a peaceful atmosphere during labor. Use headphones or speakers to play your favorite music playlist or relaxation tracks that help you stay focused and calm during contractions.

Acupressure and Reflexology: Explore acupressure and reflexology techniques to stimulate specific pressure points on the body that may help alleviate pain and promote relaxation during labor. Work with a trained practitioner or learn self-administered acupressure techniques to target areas associated with pain relief and comfort.

Hypnosis and Hypnotherapy: Consider using hypnosis or hypnotherapy techniques to induce a state of deep relaxation, reduce anxiety, and manage pain during labor. Practice self-hypnosis, guided imagery, or hypnobirthing techniques to enter a trance-like state and enhance your ability to cope with labor pain.

t's important to remember that coping mechanisms for labor pain are highly ndividualized, and what works for one woman may not work for another. Explore lifferent techniques, experiment with various coping strategies, and trust your instincts to find what feels most effective and comfortable for you during VBAC labor. Additionally, work closely with your healthcare provider, labor support team, and birth partner to develop a personalized pain management plan that meets your needs and preferences for childbirth.

Understanding the stages of labor and VBAC-specific considerations

Understanding the stages of labor is essential for women planning Vaginal Birth After Cesarean (VBAC), as it helps them prepare for the progression of childbirth and make informed decisions about their care. VBAC-specific considerations may affect how labor unfolds and impact the management of each stage. Here's an overview of the stages of labor and VBAC-specific considerations:

1. Early Labor:

Definition: Early labor, also known as the latent phase, is the initial stage of labor characterized by mild contractions that gradually increase in frequency, duration, and intensity. Cervical dilation begins, but progress may be slow and irregular.

VBAC Considerations: In VBAC, early labor may progress differently than in first-time pregnancies or repeat cesarean deliveries. Women with a history of cesarean delivery may experience variations in cervical readiness and labor progression due to factors such as uterine scar integrity and pelvic dynamics. Monitoring for signs of uterine rupture or scar dehiscence is essential during early labor in VBAC.

2. Active Labor:

Definition: Active labor is the phase of labor when cervical dilation accelerates, and contractions become stronger, longer, and more frequent. Cervical dilation progresses to approximately 6-7 centimeters.

VBAC Considerations: Active labor may proceed similarly in VBAC as in other types of childbirth, but vigilance for signs of uterine rupture or scar complications is crucial. Continuous fetal monitoring, close observation of labor progress, and readiness for prompt intervention in the event of complications are important aspects of VBAC management during active labor.

. Transition:

Definition: Transition is the shortest and most intense phase of labor, characterized by rapid cervical dilation from approximately 8-10 centimeters. Contractions reach peak intensity, and the urge to push may become overwhelming.

VBAC Considerations: Transition in VBAC may present unique challenges and considerations due to the potential for scar-related complications. Healthcare providers must be prepared to manage emergent situations such as uterine rupture promptly. Continuous fetal monitoring, close observation of maternal and fetal well-being, and readiness for operative delivery if needed are essential during transition in VBAC.

4. Pushing and Delivery:

Definition: The pushing stage of labor occurs when the cervix is fully dilated (10 centimeters), and the woman begins actively pushing to facilitate the baby's descent through the birth canal. Delivery occurs when the baby's head emerges from the vagina, followed by the rest of the body.

VBAC Considerations: Pushing and delivery in VBAC may proceed similarly to other types of childbirth, but careful monitoring for signs of uterine rupture or scar complications is necessary. Healthcare providers should be prepared to intervene promptly if complications arise and may consider alternative delivery methods, such as vacuum extraction or forceps, depending on the clinical situation.

Understanding the stages of labor and VBAC-specific considerations empowers women and healthcare providers to navigate childbirth safely and effectively. Continuous monitoring, individualized care, and readiness for prompt intervention are essential components of VBAC management throughout each stage of labor. By staying informed and proactive, women planning VBAC can work collaboratively with their healthcare team to achieve a positive and empowering childbirth experience while prioritizing maternal and fetal safety.

The role of the support team during labor

The support team plays a crucial role during labor for Vaginal Birth After Cesarean (VBAC), providing emotional, physical, and informational support to the birthing person and ensuring a safe and positive childbirth experience. Here's an overview of the roles and responsibilities of the support team during VBAC labor:

1. Partner or Spouse:

Emotional Support: The partner or spouse offers continuous emotional support, encouragement, and reassurance throughout labor. They provide comfort, empathy, and a sense of security to the birthing person, helping to reduce anxiety and stress.

Physical Support: Partners may assist with position changes, massage, counterpressure, and other comfort measures to alleviate labor pain and discomfort. They play an active role in supporting the birthing person's physical needs and promoting relaxation and comfort during labor.

Advocate: Partners advocate for the birthing person's preferences, wishes, and concerns during labor, communicating with healthcare providers and ensuring that the birthing person's voice is heard and respected. They participate in decision-making and help navigate any challenges or interventions that may arise during VBAC labor.

2. Doula:

Continuous Support: Doulas provide continuous physical, emotional, and informational support to the birthing person and their partner throughout labor. They offer personalized care, comfort measures, and coping strategies to help manage labor pain and promote relaxation and comfort.

Education and Guidance: Doulas offer evidence-based information, guidance, and reassurance to the birthing person and their partner, empowering them to make informed decisions about their care during VBAC labor. They provide education on VBAC-specific considerations, labor progress, pain management options, and birth preferences.

Advocacy: Doulas advocate for the birthing person's preferences and autonomy during labor, ensuring that their voice is heard and respected by healthcare providers. They help facilitate communication, navigate decision-making, and promote shared decision-making between the birthing person and their healthcare team.

3. Healthcare Providers:

Monitoring and Assessment: Obstetricians, midwives, and nurses monitor the progress of labor, assess maternal and fetal well-being, and provide medical care and interventions as needed. They conduct regular evaluations, monitor vital signs, and assess labor progress, ensuring the safety and well-being of both the birthing person and the baby.

Clinical Management: Healthcare providers oversee the clinical management of VBAC labor, including monitoring for signs of uterine rupture, scar integrity, and fetal distress. They make evidence-based decisions regarding pain management, labor augmentation, and the timing and mode of delivery, prioritizing maternal and fetal safety while respecting the birthing person's preferences and autonomy.

Communication: Healthcare providers communicate with the birthing person, their partner, and other members of the support team throughout labor, providing updates, guidance, and explanations of procedures or interventions. They foster a collaborative and supportive environment, encouraging open communication and shared decision-making.

4. Additional Support Personnel:

Hospital Staff: Labor and delivery nurses, obstetricians, midwives, and other hospital staff play integral roles in supporting VBAC labor. They provide medical care, assist with labor management, and ensure a safe and supportive environment for childbirth.

Family Members or Friends: Additional family members or friends may offer emotional support, assistance, and encouragement to the birthing person and their partner during VBAC labor. Their presence can provide comfort and companionship during the birthing process.

The support team collaborates closely to create a supportive and empowering environment for VBAC labor, ensuring that the birthing person feels safe, respected, and supported throughout the childbirth journey. By working together, the support team helps facilitate a positive and memorable VBAC experience while prioritizing maternal and fetal well-being.

Making informed decisions during labor for Vaginal Birth After Cesarean (VBAC) is crucial for ensuring the safety, well-being, and satisfaction of the birthing person and their baby. Here's a guide to making informed decisions during VBAC labor:

1. Understand Your Options:

Know Your Birth Preferences: Before labor begins, clarify your preferences, values, and goals for VBAC. Consider factors such as pain management preferences, labor interventions, movement and positioning during labor, and preferences for delivery.

Learn About VBAC-Specific Considerations: Educate yourself about VBAC-specific considerations, including the risks and benefits of VBAC compared to repeat cesarean delivery, factors influencing VBAC success, and potential complications such as uterine rupture.

Discuss Pain Management Options: Explore various pain management options available during VBAC labor, including pharmacological and non-pharmacological interventions. Learn about the benefits, risks, and alternatives to pain relief methods to make informed decisions about pain management.

.. Communicate with Your Healthcare Team:

Establish Open Communication: Build a trusting relationship with your healthcare providers, including obstetricians, midwives, nurses, and doulas. Establish open communication channels to discuss your preferences, concerns, and questions about VBAC labor.

Ask Questions: Don't hesitate to ask questions and seek clarification about VBAC-related topics, labor progress, interventions, and potential complications. Request evidence-based information and explanations from your healthcare providers to help you make informed decisions.

Discuss Risks and Benefits: Engage in discussions with your healthcare team about the risks and benefits of VBAC, including potential complications such as uterine rupture, scar dehiscence, and the likelihood of successful vaginal birth based on your individual circumstances.

3. Stay Informed and Involved:

Stay Educated: Stay informed about the progress of labor, including cervical dilation, fetal heart rate monitoring, and any interventions or procedures recommended by your healthcare team. Ask for updates and explanations about any changes or developments during labor.

Participate in Decision-Making: Take an active role in decision-making during labor, considering your preferences, values, and the best interests of you and your baby. Collaborate with your healthcare team to weigh the benefits and risks of interventions and make decisions that align with your birth plan and goals.

Request Time to Consider Options: If faced with a decision during labor, such as the need for labor augmentation, pain medication, or cesarean delivery, request time to consider your options, gather information, and discuss with your partner and healthcare providers before making a decision.

4. Trust Your Instincts:

Listen to Your Body: Trust your instincts and listen to your body's signals during labor. Pay attention to your comfort level, pain tolerance, and intuition about what feels right for you and your baby.

Be Flexible: While it's essential to have a birth plan and preferences for VBAC labor, be prepared to adapt and make changes based on the evolving circumstances of labor. Stay flexible and open-minded about interventions or changes to the birth plan that may be necessary for the safety and well-being of you and your baby.

5. Advocate for Yourself:

Assert Your Preferences: Advocate for your preferences, wishes, and concerns during labor, expressing your needs clearly and assertively to your healthcare providers. Use "I" statements to communicate your desires and preferences respectfully and confidently.

Seek a Second Opinion: If you have reservations or uncertainties about a recommended intervention or decision during labor, consider seeking a second opinion from another healthcare provider or consulting with a trusted advocate or support person.

6. Have a Supportive Birth Team:

Surround Yourself with Support: Surround yourself with a supportive birth team, including your partner, doula, family members, or friends who can offer encouragement, guidance, and advocacy during VBAC labor. Seek emotional support and reassurance from your support team as you navigate labor and make decisions.

By staying informed, communicating openly with your healthcare team, actively participating in decision-making, and trusting your instincts, you can make informed decisions during VBAC labor that promote a safe, satisfying, and empowering childbirth experience for you and your baby. Remember that every labor experience is unique, and prioritizing informed decision-making helps you advocate for your preferences and well-being throughout the VBAC journey.

Emergency scenarios and contingency plans

Preparing for emergency scenarios and having contingency plans in place is essential for Vaginal Birth After Cesarean (VBAC) to ensure the safety and well-being of the birthing person and their baby. While VBAC is generally considered safe, there is a small risk of complications such as uterine rupture, which requires prompt recognition and management. Here are some emergency scenarios and contingency plans for VBAC:

1. Uterine Rupture:

Recognition: Healthcare providers monitor for signs and symptoms of uterine rupture during labor, including abnormal fetal heart rate patterns, sudden onset of severe abdominal pain, vaginal bleeding, and changes in uterine contractions. Continuous fetal monitoring is essential for early detection of fetal distress.

Management: If uterine rupture is suspected or confirmed, immediate intervention is necessary. Healthcare providers may initiate emergency measures such as cesarean delivery, blood transfusion, and resuscitation as needed. Surgical repair of the uterine rupture may be required to control bleeding and ensure maternal and fetal safety.

2. Scar Dehiscence:

Recognition: Scar dehiscence refers to separation or reopening of the uterine scar from a previous cesarean delivery without full uterine rupture. It may present with symptoms similar to uterine rupture, including abdominal pain, vaginal bleeding, and changes in fetal heart rate patterns.

Management: Scar dehiscence may be managed conservatively or surgically, depending on the extent of the separation and the clinical condition of the birthing person and the baby. Healthcare providers closely monitor maternal and fetal well-being and may consider cesarean delivery if there are concerns about uterine integrity or fetal distress.

3. Fetal Distress:

Recognition: Fetal distress may occur during labor due to factors such as umbilical cord compression, placental insufficiency, or other complications. Healthcare providers monitor fetal heart rate patterns for signs of distress, including persistent tachycardia, bradycardia, late decelerations, or variable decelerations.

Management: If fetal distress is suspected or confirmed, healthcare providers take immediate action to optimize maternal and fetal well-being. This may include repositioning the birthing person, providing oxygen supplementation, administering intravenous fluids, or preparing for expedited delivery, such as assisted vaginal delivery or cesarean section, depending on the severity of the situation.

4. Maternal Hemorrhage:

Recognition: Maternal hemorrhage is a life-threatening complication characterized by excessive bleeding during or after childbirth. Healthcare providers monitor for signs of hemorrhage, such as persistent vaginal bleeding, hypotension, tachycardia, or signs of shock.

Management: Prompt recognition and management of maternal hemorrhage are critical for preventing complications and ensuring maternal survival. Healthcare providers initiate interventions such as uterine massage, administration of uterotonic medications, and surgical intervention if necessary to control bleeding and stabilize the birthing person's condition.

5. Failed VBAC:

Recognition: In some cases, VBAC may not progress as planned, leading to a failed trial of labor. This may occur due to factors such as stalled labor, fetal distress, maternal exhaustion, or other complications.

Management: If VBAC is unsuccessful, healthcare providers may recommend cesarean delivery to ensure the safety of the birthing person and the baby. A failed VBAC does not necessarily preclude future attempts at vaginal birth, but individualized assessment and planning are necessary to minimize risks and optimize outcomes in subsequent pregnancies.

. Neonatal Resuscitation:

Recognition: In rare cases, neonatal resuscitation may be required immediately after birth due to factors such as meconium aspiration, birth trauma, or fetal distress during labor.

Management: Healthcare providers trained in neonatal resuscitation techniques initiate appropriate interventions to support the newborn's transition to extrauterine life. This may include suctioning of the airway, positive pressure ventilation, chest compressions, administration of medications, and other measures as needed to stabilize the baby's condition.

7. Communication and Coordination:

Effective Communication: Clear communication and coordination among members of the healthcare team are essential for recognizing, managing, and resolving emergency scenarios during VBAC labor. Healthcare providers communicate openly with the birthing person and their support team, providing updates, explanations, and guidance throughout the process.

Emergency Protocols: Healthcare facilities have established emergency protocols and procedures for managing obstetric emergencies, including VBAC-related complications. Healthcare providers are trained to implement these protocols swiftly and effectively to optimize outcomes and ensure the safety of the birthing person and the baby.

8. Shared Decision-Making:

Informed Consent: In emergency scenarios, healthcare providers engage in shared decision-making with the birthing person and their support team, providing information, explanations, and options for care. Informed consent is obtained before initiating any interventions or procedures, and the birthing person's preferences and autonomy are respected throughout the decision-making process.

Respect for Preferences: Healthcare providers consider the birthing person's preferences, values, and wishes when making decisions about emergency management, ensuring that care is individualized, respectful, and aligned with the birthing person's goals for childbirth.

9. Continuity of Care:

Continuity of Care: Continuity of care is maintained throughout VBAC labor, with consistent monitoring, assessment, and support from healthcare providers and the birthing person's support team. Regular communication and collaboration ensure a seamless transition between stages of labor and facilitate optimal management of emergency scenarios.

10. Postpartum Follow-Up:

Postpartum Monitoring: After childbirth, healthcare providers conduct postpartum monitoring and assessment to ensure the birthing person's recovery and well-being. This may include monitoring for signs of postpartum hemorrhage, uterine involution, breastfeeding support, and emotional support for the birthing person and their family.

Immediate postpartum care after VBAC

Immediate postpartum care after Vaginal Birth After Cesarean (VBAC) is crucial for ensuring the well-being of the birthing person and their baby, promoting recovery, and addressing any potential complications that may arise. Here are key aspects of immediate postpartum care after VBAC:

1. Maternal Assessment:

Vital Signs Monitoring: Healthcare providers monitor the birthing person's vital signs, including blood pressure, heart rate, and temperature, to assess for signs of hemorrhage, infection, or other complications.

Uterine Assessment: Healthcare providers assess uterine tone, fundal height, and lochia (postpartum bleeding) to ensure adequate contraction of the uterus and address any concerns regarding uterine atony or excessive bleeding.

Perineal Care: Healthcare providers assess the perineum for lacerations, tears, or episiotomy and provide appropriate care, including pain relief, perineal hygiene, and wound management.

2. Neonatal Care:

Immediate Assessment: Healthcare providers conduct a thorough assessment of the newborn, including Apgar scoring, assessment of breathing, heart rate, muscle tone, reflexes, and skin color, to ensure the baby's well-being and identify any immediate concerns.

Skin-to-Skin Contact: Encourage skin-to-skin contact between the birthing person and the newborn to promote bonding, warmth, breastfeeding initiation, and stabilization of the baby's vital signs.

Breastfeeding Support: Offer breastfeeding support and assistance to the birthing person, including guidance on positioning, latch techniques, and early breastfeeding initiation to establish breastfeeding and promote milk production.

3. Pain Management:

Pain Assessment: Healthcare providers assess the birthing person's pain level and provide appropriate pain management interventions, including pharmacological and non-pharmacological methods, to alleviate discomfort and promote recovery.

Medication Administration: Administer pain medications as prescribed or requested by the birthing person, considering individual preferences, allergies, and medical history. Offer options such as nonsteroidal anti-inflammatory drugs (NSAIDs), acetaminophen, or opioid analgesics as needed.

4. Emotional Support:

Psychological Assessment: Assess the birthing person's emotional well-being and provide emotional support, reassurance, and validation of their experience. Address any concerns, fears, or anxieties related to childbirth, postpartum recovery, or caring for a newborn.

Encourage Bonding: Encourage bonding and interaction between the birthing person, their partner, and the newborn, fostering a nurturing and supportive environment for the family unit.

5. Monitoring for Complications:

Hemorrhage Prevention: Monitor the birthing person for signs of postpartum hemorrhage, including excessive bleeding, uterine atony, and signs of shock. Promptly intervene with uterotonic medications, uterine massage, or other measures to control bleeding and stabilize the birthing person's condition.

Infection Prevention: Monitor for signs of infection, including fever, abdominal pain, foul-smelling lochia, or signs of wound infection. Implement infection prevention measures, including hand hygiene, sterile technique for wound care, and administration of prophylactic antibiotics as indicated.

6. Education and Discharge Planning:

Postpartum Education: Provide comprehensive education to the birthing person and their support team on postpartum recovery, newborn care, breastfeeding, contraception, and signs of postpartum complications. Address any questions or concerns and provide written materials or resources for reference.

Discharge Planning: Develop a discharge plan in collaboration with the birthing person, including instructions for postpartum care, follow-up appointments, and contact information for healthcare providers. Ensure that the birthing person feels confident and prepared to manage their postpartum recovery and newborn care at home.

7. Follow-Up Care:

Postpartum Follow-Up: Schedule follow-up appointments for the birthing person and newborn to monitor recovery, assess breastfeeding progress, and address any postpartum concerns or complications. Provide ongoing support and guidance to promote optimal maternal and newborn health during the postpartum period.

By providing comprehensive immediate postpartum care after VBAC, healthcare providers can optimize outcomes, support recovery, and promote the well-being of the birthing person and their newborn. Effective communication, individualized care, and proactive management of complications are essential components of postpartum care for VBAC.

Breastfeeding and bonding with your baby

Breastfeeding and bonding with your baby after Vaginal Birth After Cesarean (VBAC) are important aspects of postpartum recovery and early parenting. Here's how you can promote breastfeeding and bonding after VBAC:

1. Early Initiation of Breastfeeding:

Skin-to-Skin Contact: Initiate skin-to-skin contact between you and your baby as soon as possible after birth, ideally within the first hour. Skin-to-skin contact help regulate your baby's temperature, heart rate, and breathing, and promotes bonding and breastfeeding initiation.

Breastfeeding Cue Recognition: Learn to recognize your baby's early feeding cues such as rooting, sucking motions, and hand-to-mouth movements, to initiate breastfeeding when your baby is ready.

Latch Assistance: Seek assistance from healthcare providers, lactation consultants, or breastfeeding support personnel to ensure a proper latch and comfortable breastfeeding position for you and your baby.

2. Supportive Breastfeeding Environment:

Encourage Rooming-In: If possible, opt for rooming-in with your baby to promote frequent breastfeeding and bonding opportunities. Having your baby close by allows for more frequent feeding sessions and enhances the parent-infant bond.

Access to Resources: Take advantage of available resources and support services for breastfeeding, such as lactation consultants, breastfeeding support groups, and educational materials. Seek guidance and assistance as needed to overcome breastfeeding challenges and establish a successful breastfeeding relationship.

3. Bonding Activities:

Eye Contact and Touch: Engage in frequent eye contact, gentle touch, and skin-to-skin cuddling with your baby to promote bonding and emotional connection. Bonding activities such as talking, singing, and caressing your baby enhance the parent-infant relationship and promote feelings of closeness and attachment.

Responsive Caregiving: Respond promptly to your baby's cues and needs, including hunger, comfort, and soothing. Providing responsive caregiving fosters trust and security and strengthens the bond between you and your baby.

4. Breastfeeding Benefits:

Health Benefits: Breastfeeding offers numerous health benefits for both you and your baby, including protection against infections, enhanced immune function, and optimal nutrition. Breastfeeding also promotes bonding and emotional connection between you and your baby.

Bonding Hormones: Breastfeeding stimulates the release of hormones such as oxytocin, often referred to as the "love hormone," which enhances feelings of maternal attachment and bonding. Nursing sessions provide opportunities for intimate connection and nurturing interaction between you and your baby.

5. Patience and Persistence:

Be Patient: Be patient with yourself and your baby as you navigate the breastfeeding journey together. Breastfeeding may take time to establish, and both you and your baby may need time to learn and adjust to the breastfeeding process.

Seek Support: Don't hesitate to seek support and guidance from healthcare providers, lactation consultants, or peer support groups if you encounter challenges or concerns with breastfeeding. Supportive assistance can help troubleshoot issues, provide encouragement, and enhance your breastfeeding experience.

6. Self-Care:

Take Care of Yourself: Prioritize self-care and well-being as you adjust to the demands of breastfeeding and postpartum recovery. Get adequate rest, nutrition, and hydration, and enlist support from family members or friends to assist with household tasks and childcare responsibilities.

Emotional Support: Reach out for emotional support if you're experiencing feelings of overwhelm, stress, or postpartum mood disorders. Connect with trusted support persons, healthcare providers, or mental health professionals for guidance and assistance.

Breastfeeding and bonding after VBAC are precious opportunities to nurture your baby's growth and development while fostering a strong and loving connection between you and your little one. By prioritizing skin-to-skin contact, responsive caregiving, and access to breastfeeding support, you can establish a fulfilling breastfeeding relationship and build a deep bond with your baby that lasts a lifetime.

Physical recovery after VBAC compared to cesarean section

Physical recovery after Vaginal Birth After Cesarean (VBAC) and cesarean section (C-section) can vary based on individual circumstances, including the birthing person's overall health, the presence of any complications during childbirth, and the mode of delivery. Here's a comparison of physical recovery after VBAC and cesarean section:

Physical Recovery After VBAC:

Vaginal Birth: In VBAC, the birthing person delivers the baby vaginally, which typically results in less trauma to the abdominal muscles and tissues compared to cesarean delivery. Recovery may be faster and involve fewer postoperative complications such as wound infections or incisional pain.

Less Pain: Many individuals who have a VBAC experience less postpartum pain compared to those who undergo cesarean delivery. Vaginal birth is associated with fewer incision-related discomforts and may allow for earlier mobility and activity.

Shorter Hospital Stay: In many cases, individuals who have a VBAC experience a shorter hospital stay compared to those who undergo cesarean delivery. With an uncomplicated VBAC, individuals may be discharged home sooner, allowing for a quicker return to the comfort of their own environment.

Faster Return to Normal Activities: Because VBAC typically involves less extensive surgical recovery, individuals may resume normal activities such as walking, lifting, and caring for themselves and their baby more quickly than after a cesarean section.

Lower Risk of Surgical Complications: VBAC is associated with a lower risk of surgical complications such as wound infections, adhesions, and incisional hernias compared to repeat cesarean delivery. The absence of abdominal surgery reduces the likelihood of postoperative complications related to the surgical incision.

Physical Recovery After Cesarean Section:

Surgical Recovery: Cesarean section involves abdominal surgery to deliver the baby, resulting in longer and potentially more challenging physical recovery compared to vaginal birth. The birthing person may experience postoperative pain, discomfort, and limited mobility during the initial recovery period.

Incision Care: Individuals who undergo cesarean delivery require meticulous care of the surgical incision to prevent infection, promote healing, and minimize scarring. Proper wound care, including keeping the incision clean and dry, avoiding strenuous activities, and following healthcare provider instructions, is essential for optimal recovery.

Pain Management: Cesarean delivery often involves greater postpartum pain compared to vaginal birth, particularly during the first few days after surgery. Pain management strategies such as medications, ice packs, and positioning aids may be necessary to alleviate discomfort and promote recovery.

Restricted Activities: Following cesarean delivery, individuals may need to restrict certain activities such as heavy lifting, driving, and strenuous exercise for several weeks to allow the surgical incision to heal properly. Limiting physical exertion and practicing good body mechanics can help prevent complications and promote optimal recovery.

Longer Hospital Stay: Cesarean delivery typically requires a longer hospital stay compared to vaginal birth, particularly if there are complications or additional monitoring needed for the birthing person or baby. Extended hospitalization may impact postpartum recovery and adjustment to parenthood.

Increased Risk of Complications: Cesarean delivery carries a higher risk of surgical complications such as wound infections, blood clots, and adhesions compared to vaginal birth. Individuals who undergo cesarean section may require ongoing monitoring and follow-up care to address any postoperative complications that arise.

It's important to note that every birthing experience is unique, and individual factors such as overall health, personal preferences, and birth outcomes can influence the physical recovery process after VBAC or cesarean section. Healthcare providers work closely with birthing individuals to provide personalized care, support, and guidance throughout the postpartum period to optimize recovery and promote well-being.

Emotional support for both partners during the postpartum period for an unsuccessful VBAC

Experiencing a failed Vaginal Birth After Cesarean (VBAC) can be emotionally challenging for both partners during the postpartum period. It's essential to provide mutual support, understanding, and empathy to navigate this experience together. Here are some ways to offer emotional support for both partners:

1. Open Communication:

Express Feelings: Encourage open and honest communication between partners about their feelings, thoughts, and reactions to the failed VBAC. Create a safe space where both partners feel comfortable sharing their emotions without judgment or criticism.

Active Listening: Practice active listening by attentively hearing and validating each other's perspectives. Allow each partner to express their concerns, disappointments, and fears, and offer empathetic responses and reassurance.

2. Validate Emotions:

Normalize Feelings: Recognize that feelings of disappointment, sadness, anger, or frustration are normal and valid responses to a failed VBAC. Validate each other's emotions and reassure one another that it's okay to grieve the loss of the desired birth experience.

Empathize: Show empathy and understanding toward each other's emotional experiences. Acknowledge the impact of the failed VBAC on both partners and offer comfort and support during moments of vulnerability.

3. Seek Support:

Professional Counseling: Consider seeking support from a mental health professional, counselor, or therapist who specializes in perinatal mental health. Professional counseling can provide a safe and supportive environment to explore emotions, develop coping strategies, and navigate the complexities of the failed VBAC experience.

Support Groups: Joining a support group for individuals who have experienced a failed VBAC or perinatal loss can offer peer support, validation, and solidarity. Connecting with others who share similar experiences can reduce feelings of isolation and provide a sense of community and understanding.

4. Focus on Healing:

Self-Care: Prioritize self-care practices for both partners to promote emotional well-being and resilience. Encourage activities such as exercise, relaxation techniques, hobbies, and social connections that nourish and rejuvenate the mind and body.

Quality Time Together: Carve out quality time to nurture your relationship and bond as partners outside of the challenges of the failed VBAC experience. Engage in activities that bring joy, laughter, and connection, such as spending time outdoors, watching movies, or enjoying meals together.

5. Maintain Perspective:

Focus on What Went Right: Encourage each other to focus on the positives and accomplishments during childbirth, regardless of the outcome. Celebrate the strength, courage, and resilience demonstrated by both partners throughout the birthing process.

Hope and Future Planning: Maintain optimism and hope for the future, recognizing that the failed VBAC is just one chapter in your journey as a family. Discuss future plans, goals, and aspirations together, and explore options for future pregnancies and birth experiences with the support of healthcare providers.

5. Be Patient and Gentle:

Practice Patience: Be patient and understanding with each other as you navigate the emotional aftermath of the failed VBAC. Recognize that healing takes time, and allow space for each partner to process emotions and move forward at their own pace.

Offer Gentleness: Approach each other with kindness, compassion, and gentleness as you support one another through the ups and downs of the postpartum period. Offer words of affirmation, acts of kindness, and gestures of love to nurture your bond and strengthen your connection as partners.

By providing mutual emotional support, validation, and understanding, partners can navigate the challenges of a failed VBAC together and emerge stronger, more resilient, and more connected as a couple. Remember that seeking professional support and prioritizing self-care are essential components of coping with the emotional impact of the failed VBAC and promoting overall well-being for both partners.

Adjusting to life with a newborn after VBAC

Long-term health considerations for both mother and baby after VBAC

Chapter 8: Advocating for VBAC Rights and Resources

Understanding your rights surrounding VBAC

Adjusting to life with a newborn after Vaginal Birth After Cesarean (VBAC) involves navigating the physical, emotional, and practical aspects of newborn care while recovering from childbirth. Here are some tips to help both partners adjust to life with a newborn after VBAC:

1. Prioritize Self-Care:

Rest and Sleep: Prioritize rest and sleep whenever possible, taking turns with your partner to care for the baby and allowing each other to rest. Nap when the baby sleeps to replenish energy levels and promote physical recovery.

Nutrition: Maintain a healthy diet rich in nutritious foods to support your postpartum recovery and breastfeeding journey. Stay hydrated and nourished to sustain your energy levels and promote overall well-being.

Emotional Wellness: Take care of your emotional well-being by seeking support from your partner, family members, friends, or healthcare providers. Practice self-compassion, and be gentle with yourself as you navigate the challenges and joys of parenthood.

2. Establish Routines and Rituals:

Create Predictable Routines: Establish predictable routines for feeding, diapering, sleeping, and bonding with your baby. Consistent routines can help both partners feel more confident and competent in caring for the newborn and promote a sense of stability during the postpartum period.

Share Responsibilities: Divide caregiving responsibilities with your partner, taking turns with tasks such as feeding, diaper changes, soothing, and bedtime routines. Collaborative caregiving fosters teamwork and strengthens your bond as partners and parents.

3. Communicate Effectively:

Open Communication: Maintain open and honest communication with your partner about your needs, concerns, and experiences as new parents. Discuss parenting strategies, preferences, and goals together, and work as a team to address challenges and make decisions that are best for your family.

Express Gratitude: Express appreciation and gratitude for your partner's support, contributions, and efforts in caring for the newborn and managing household responsibilities. Acknowledge each other's strengths and celebrate small victories together as you navigate parenthood.

4. Seek Support and Resources:

Reach Out for Help: Don't hesitate to ask for help from family members, friends, or community resources if you need assistance with newborn care, household chores, or emotional support. Accept offers of help graciously and prioritize self-care to avoid burnout.

Utilize Healthcare Services: Take advantage of healthcare services such as postpartum check-ups, lactation support, and newborn care consultations to address any concerns or questions you may have about your baby's health and development. Trust your healthcare providers as valuable sources of guidance and support.

5. Foster Bonding and Connection:

Skin-to-Skin Contact: Maximize opportunities for skin-to-skin contact and bonding with your baby, promoting feelings of closeness, security, and attachment. Spend quality time cuddling, talking, singing, and engaging in gentle touch to strengthen your bond as parents.

Involve Your Partner: Encourage your partner to actively participate in bonding activities with the baby, such as bathing, diapering, babywearing, and playtime. Sharing caregiving responsibilities fosters a sense of connection and cohesiveness in your parenting partnership.

6. Be Flexible and Patient:

Embrace Flexibility: Embrace flexibility and adaptability as you adjust to the unpredictable nature of newborn care. Recognize that plans may need to change, and be willing to adjust expectations and priorities based on your baby's needs and cues.

Practice Patience: Practice patience and compassion with yourself and your partner as you navigate the learning curve of parenthood. Allow yourselves grace and understanding as you grow and evolve together as parents.

7. Cherish Moments of Joy:

Celebrate Milestones: Celebrate milestones, no matter how small, and cherish precious moments of joy with your newborn. Take photographs, create keepsakes, and savor the fleeting moments of infancy as you create lasting memories together as a family.

Focus on Connection: Focus on building a strong foundation of love, trust, and connection with your baby, prioritizing moments of intimacy and bonding over perfectionism or external pressures. Trust your instincts as parents, and nurture your relationship with your baby with warmth, patience, and unconditional love.

Adjusting to life with a newborn after VBAC is a journey filled with both challenges and rewards. By prioritizing self-care, effective communication, shared responsibility, and meaningful connection, both partners can navigate the joys and trials of parenthood with esilience, grace, and love. Remember to be gentle with yourselves and each other as you

embrace the transformative experience of welcoming a new life into your family.

Overcoming barriers to VBAC access and support

Overcoming barriers to Vaginal Birth After Cesarean (VBAC) access and support is

essential to ensuring that birthing individuals have the opportunity to make informed

choices about their birth experiences and receive the appropriate care and support they

need. Here are some strategies for addressing common barriers to VBAC access and

support:

1. Education and Awareness:

Community Education: Provide education and information about VBAC options,

benefits, risks, and evidence-based practices to healthcare providers, birthing

individuals, and community members. Raise awareness about the safety and

feasibility of VBAC for eligible candidates and dispel myths and misconceptions

surrounding VBAC.

Prenatal Education: Offer comprehensive prenatal education classes that cover

VBAC-specific topics, including the physiology of childbirth, labor management,

pain management options, and decision-making processes. Empower birthing individuals to advocate for their preferences and make informed decisions about

VBAC.

2. Accessible Healthcare Services:

Provider Training: Offer continuing education and training programs for

healthcare providers, including obstetricians, midwives, nurses, and doulas, on

VBAC guidelines, protocols, and best practices. Ensure that healthcare providers

are knowledgeable, skilled, and supportive of VBAC as a viable option for eligible

individuals.

Availability of VBAC-Friendly Providers: Increase access to VBAC-friendly

healthcare providers who are experienced in supporting VBAC and have a

collaborative approach to care. Expand options for birthing individuals to choose

providers who respect their preferences and offer personalized, evidence-based

care.

3. Individualized Care Planning:

Shared Decision-Making: Implement shared decision-making models that involve

birthing individuals in the decision-making process about their birth preferences,

including VBAC options. Provide comprehensive counseling and support to help

individuals weigh the benefits, risks, and alternatives to VBAC based on their

individual circumstances and preferences.

Tailored Care Plans: Develop individualized care plans for birthing individuals considering VBAC, taking into account their medical history, obstetric risk factors, preferences, and values. Collaborate with birthing individuals to develop personalized birth plans that reflect their goals and priorities for childbirth.

4. Supportive Policies and Practices:

Hospital Policies: Review and revise hospital policies and practices related to VBAC to ensure that they support evidence-based care and respect the autonomy and choices of birthing individuals. Encourage hospitals to adopt policies that promote VBAC access, including trial of labor after cesarean (TOLAC) and supportive labor management practices.

Insurance Coverage: Advocate for comprehensive insurance coverage for VBAC-related services, including prenatal care, childbirth education, labor support, and postpartum care. Ensure that insurance policies do not impose unnecessary restrictions or barriers to VBAC access and reimbursement for healthcare providers.

5. Addressing Stigma and Bias:

Combat Stigmatization: Challenge stigmatizing attitudes, biases, and stereotypes surrounding VBAC within healthcare settings, communities, and social networks.

Promote respectful language and attitudes that honor birthing individuals' autonomy, agency, and choices regarding childbirth.

Cultural Competency: Provide cultural competency training for healthcare providers to address cultural beliefs, values, and preferences related to childbirth, including VBAC. Ensure that care providers recognize and respect diverse cultural perspectives on childbirth and support birthing individuals in their decision-making process.

6. Community Support and Advocacy:

Peer Support Networks: Establish peer support networks, online forums, and community groups for individuals considering VBAC, as well as those who have experienced VBAC or cesarean birth. Create opportunities for peer-to-peer support, sharing of experiences, and emotional validation within a supportive and nonjudgmental environment.

Advocacy Efforts: Engage in advocacy efforts at local, regional, and national levels to promote VBAC access and support, including policy initiatives, legislative advocacy, public awareness campaigns, and grassroots organizing. Collaborate with stakeholders, advocacy organizations, and policymakers to address systemic barriers and improve VBAC access for all birthing individuals.

By addressing barriers to VBAC access and support through education, advocacy, policy changes, and cultural shifts within healthcare systems and communities, we can empower birthing individuals to make informed choices about their childbirth experiences and receive the respectful, personalized care they deserve.

Finding community and support networks for VBAC advocacy

Finding community and support networks for Vaginal Birth After Cesarean (VBAC) advocacy can provide invaluable resources, guidance, and solidarity for individuals passionate about promoting VBAC access and support. Here are some ways to connect with VBAC advocacy communities and support networks:

1. Online Forums and Social Media Groups:

VBAC Support Groups: Join online forums, social media groups, and virtual communities specifically dedicated to VBAC advocacy and support. Platforms such as Facebook, Reddit, and online forums like VBAC.com and The VBAC Link provide spaces for individuals to connect, share experiences, ask questions, and access resources related to VBAC advocacy.

Hashtags: Follow relevant hashtags such as #VBAC, #VBACsupport, and #VBACadvocacy on social media platforms like Instagram and Twitter to discover posts, articles, and discussions related to VBAC advocacy and support.

2. Local Support Groups and Meetups:

Local Birth Networks: Connect with local birth networks, childbirth education classes, and maternal health organizations in your community that may offer support groups, meetups, or events focused on VBAC advocacy and support. Attend meetings, workshops, or gatherings to connect with like-minded individuals and share experiences.

Doula and Midwifery Networks: Reach out to doulas, midwives, and birth professionals in your area who are supportive of VBAC and inquire about any local support groups or networking opportunities they may offer for individuals interested in VBAC advocacy.

3. Online Webinars and Workshops:

Virtual Events: Participate in online webinars, workshops, and conferences organized by VBAC advocacy organizations, childbirth educators, and maternal health professionals. These virtual events may cover topics such as VBAC rights, informed decision-making, birth justice, and policy advocacy related to VBAC access.

Professional Organizations: Explore membership in professional organizations such as the International Cesarean Awareness Network (ICAN) , The Doula

Group, and the VBAC Link, which offer resources, webinars, and networking opportunities for individuals involved in VBAC advocacy and support.

4. Advocacy Organizations and Resources:

ICAN Chapters: Get involved with local chapters of the International Cesarean Awareness Network (ICAN), which advocate for evidence-based maternity care, VBAC access, and cesarean prevention. Participate in chapter meetings, events, and advocacy campaigns to support VBAC rights and awareness in your community.

Resource Websites: Explore websites and online resources dedicated to VBAC advocacy and support, such as VBAC.com, The VBAC Link, and Evidence Based Birth. These websites offer information, toolkits, fact sheets, and advocacy resources for individuals interested in promoting VBAC access and education.

5. Social Activism and Grassroots Organizing:

Community Events: Attend rallies, marches, and community events focused on maternal health, reproductive rights, and birth justice. Participate in advocacy campaigns and grassroots organizing efforts to raise awareness about VBAC access, combat stigma, and promote equitable maternity care practices.

Collaborative Projects: Collaborate with local organizations, activists, and healthcare providers to initiate projects, campaigns, or initiatives that address barriers to VBAC access, such as policy advocacy, community outreach, and public education efforts.

6. Peer-to-Peer Support and Mentorship:

Mentorship Programs: Seek mentorship from individuals who have experience with VBAC advocacy and support, whether they are birth professionals, peer mentors, or community leaders. Connect with experienced advocates who can provide guidance, support, and mentorship as you navigate your own advocacy journey.

Online Mentorship Platforms: Explore online mentorship platforms or networks that facilitate connections between individuals interested in VBAC advocacy and experienced mentors in the field. Engage in peer-to-peer support, knowledge-sharing, and collaborative projects with fellow advocates.

By actively engaging with VBAC advocacy communities, support networks, and resources, individuals can contribute to the collective effort to promote VBAC access, education, and empowerment for birthing individuals and families around the world. Together, we can work towards a future where all individuals have access to respectful, evidence-based maternity care and the opportunity to make informed choices about their childbirth experiences.

Resources for further information and support on VBAC

'or further information and support on Vaginal Birth After Cesarean (VBAC), consider

:xploring the following resources:

. Websites and Online Platforms:

ICAN (International Cesarean Awareness Network): ICAN is a nonprofit

organization dedicated to promoting maternal health and cesarean prevention.

Their website offers resources, support groups, educational materials, and

advocacy opportunities related to VBAC and cesarean awareness.

https://www.ican-online.org/

The Doula Group: The Doula Group is South Carolina's Largest Doula Agency

and ha multiple doulas on staff that both support VBAC, as well a personal

VBACs. They hold a monthly meeting in support of VBAC, and are always there

to help address concerns around VBAC and getting you the right support.

thedoulagroup.com

The VBAC Link: The VBAC Link provides evidence-based information, online

courses, support groups, and resources for individuals considering VBAC, as well

as healthcare providers and birth professionals.https://www.thevbaclink.com/

Evidence Based Birth: Evidence Based Birth offers comprehensive articles, research summaries, podcasts, and online courses on a variety of childbirth topics, including VBAC. Their website provides evidence-based information and resources for individuals seeking informed decision-making in maternity care. Visit Evidence Based Birth

2. Books and Publications:

"The VBAC Companion: The Expectant Mother's Guide to Vaginal Birth After Cesarean" by Diana Korte and Roberta Scaer: This comprehensive guidebook provides practical information, personal stories, and expert advice on preparing for and achieving a successful VBAC.

"Birthing Normally After a Cesarean or Two" by Hélène Vadeboncoeur: This book offers insights, research, and personal experiences from women who have pursued vaginal birth after multiple cesarean deliveries.

3. Online Communities and Support Groups:

Facebook Groups: Join Facebook groups dedicated to VBAC support and advocacy, such as "VBAC Support Group," "VBAC Mama," or local VBAC support groups specific to your region.

Reddit Communities: Explore subreddits such as r/VBAC or r/BirthStories to connect with individuals sharing their experiences, questions, and resources related to VBAC.

4. Healthcare Providers and Birth Professionals:

Consult with a VBAC-Supportive Provider: Seek out obstetricians, midwives, or doulas who are experienced and supportive of VBAC. Schedule consultations to discuss your options, preferences, and concerns regarding VBAC.

VBAC-Friendly Birth Centers: Consider birthing at a VBAC-friendly birth center with healthcare providers who offer personalized, supportive care for individuals pursuing VBAC.

5. Local Birth Networks and Organizations:

Local ICAN Chapters: Connect with local chapters of the International Cesarean Awareness Network (ICAN) in your area to attend meetings, support groups, and events focused on VBAC education and advocacy.

Maternal Health Organizations: Explore local maternal health organizations, childbirth education classes, and doula collectives that may offer VBAC-specific resources, support groups, or workshops.

6. Online Courses and Workshops:

VBAC Preparation Courses: Enroll in online VBAC preparation courses or workshops that provide evidence-based information, practical tips, and emotional support for individuals considering VBAC.

By exploring these resources and connecting with supportive communities, individuals can access valuable information, guidance, and peer support to navigate their VBAC journey with confidence and empowerment. Remember to consult with trusted healthcare providers and seek personalized support that aligns with your unique needs and preferences.

How to contribute to improving VBAC access and education in your community

Contributing to improving Vaginal Birth After Cesarean (VBAC) access and education in your community is a meaningful way to advocate for evidence-based maternity care and support birthing individuals in making informed choices about their childbirth experiences. Here are some ways to contribute to VBAC access and education in your community:

1. Raise Awareness:

Host Educational Events: Organize community events, workshops, or webinars focused on VBAC education, rights, and options. Invite local healthcare providers,

VBAC advocates, and childbirth educators to share information and resources with community members.

Distribute Informational Materials: Distribute flyers, brochures, or informational packets about VBAC at local healthcare facilities, maternity clinics, libraries, and community centers. Provide evidence-based information, statistics, and resources to empower individuals with knowledge about VBAC.

2. Advocate for Policy Change:

Policy Advocacy: Advocate for policy changes at local, regional, and national levels to improve VBAC access and support. Collaborate with healthcare professionals, advocacy organizations, and policymakers to address barriers such as restrictive hospital policies, insurance coverage limitations, and provider bias against VBAC.

Legislative Initiatives: Support legislative initiatives that promote VBAC access, informed consent, and respectful maternity care practices. Write letters, make phone calls, and participate in advocacy campaigns to influence policymakers and legislators to prioritize VBAC rights and options.

3. Supportive Community Networks:

Create Support Groups: Establish local support groups or online communities for individuals considering VBAC, as well as those who have experienced VBAC or cesarean birth. Provide opportunities for peer support, sharing of experiences, and

emotional validation within a supportive and nonjudgmental environment.

Partner with Healthcare Providers: Collaborate with VBAC-friendly healthcare

providers, midwives, and doulas in your community to offer VBAC education,

counseling, and support services. Build partnerships to ensure that birthing

individuals have access to comprehensive care and resources throughout their

VBAC journey.

4. Provide Accessible Resources:

Online Resources: Develop or curate online resources, websites, and social media

platforms dedicated to VBAC education and advocacy. Offer evidence-based

information, articles, videos, and downloadable materials to support individuals in

their VBAC decision-making process.

Library Workshops: Partner with local libraries to offer workshops or information

sessions on VBAC-related topics, such as informed decision-making, birth

planning, and postpartum recovery. Provide access to books, DVDs, and other

resources about VBAC for community members to borrow.

5. Foster Collaboration and Networking:

Community Partnerships: Build collaborative partnerships with maternal health

organizations, childbirth educators, birth centers, and community groups to expand

VBAC access and education initiatives. Pool resources, share expertise, and coordinate efforts to reach a broader audience and maximize impact.

Professional Development: Offer professional development opportunities for healthcare providers, birth professionals, and childbirth educators to enhance their knowledge and skills related to VBAC support and care. Host workshops, training sessions, or continuing education programs focused on evidence-based VBAC practices and advocacy.

5. Share Personal Stories and Experiences:

Storytelling Platforms: Share personal stories, experiences, and testimonials about VBAC on social media, blogs, podcasts, and storytelling platforms. Amplify diverse voices and perspectives to raise awareness, reduce stigma, and inspire others to explore VBAC options.

Community Events: Organize storytelling events or panel discussions where individuals can share their VBAC journeys and connect with others who have similar experiences. Create opportunities for dialogue, reflection, and mutual support within the community.

By taking proactive steps to contribute to VBAC access and education in your community, you can empower birthing individuals to make informed decisions, advocate for their rights, and access the supportive care they deserve during the childbirth process.

Together, we can work towards creating a culture of respect, empowerment, and autonomy in maternity care that honors individual preferences and promotes positive birth experiences.

Appendix: Additional Resources

Recommended books, websites, and organizations for further reading and support on VBAC

Here are some recommended books, websites, and organizations for further reading and support on Vaginal Birth After Cesarean (VBAC):

Books:

"The VBAC Companion: The Expectant Mother's Guide to Vaginal Birth After Cesarean" by Diana Korte and Roberta Scaer: This comprehensive guidebook provides practical information, personal stories, and expert advice on preparing for and achieving a successful VBAC.

"Birthing Normally After a Cesarean or Two" by Hélène Vadeboncoeur: This book offers insights, research, and personal experiences from women who have pursued vaginal birth after multiple cesarean deliveries.

"VBAC: Having a Baby After a Cesarean" by Bruce K. Flamm: This book provides evidence-based information, practical tips, and personal stories to guide individuals considering VBAC through their decision-making process.

Websites:

ICAN (International Cesarean Awareness Network): ICAN is a nonprofit organization dedicated to promoting maternal health and cesarean prevention. Their website offers resources, support groups, educational materials, and advocacy opportunities related to VBAC and cesarean awareness.https://www.ican-online.org/

The VBAC Link: The VBAC Link provides evidence-based information, online courses, support groups, and resources for individuals considering VBAC, as well as healthcare providers and birth professionals.https://www.thevbaclink.com/

Evidence Based Birth: Evidence Based Birth offers comprehensive articles, research summaries, podcasts, and online courses on a variety of childbirth topics, including VBAC. Their website provides evidence-based information and resources for individuals seeking informed decision-making in maternity care.https://evidencebasedbirth.com/

Organizations:

International Cesarean Awareness Network (ICAN): ICAN is a nonprofit organization with chapters worldwide that advocate for evidence-based maternity care, VBAC access, and cesarean prevention. They offer support groups, educational resources, advocacy campaigns, and community events for individuals interested in VBAC. Find ICAN Chapters

The VBAC Project: The VBAC Project is a nonprofit organization that provides information, resources, and support for individuals considering VBAC. They offer educational materials, online forums, and advocacy efforts to promote VBAC awareness and access.https://www.thevbacproject.com/

These resources offer valuable information, support, and advocacy opportunities for individuals interested in learning more about VBAC, making informed decisions about childbirth, and accessing supportive care during the maternity journey. Explore these resources to empower yourself with knowledge, connect with supportive communities, and advocate for your birth preferences and rights.

Glossary of terms related to VBAC and childbirth

Here's a glossary of terms related to Vaginal Birth After Cesarean (VBAC) and childbirth:

VBAC (Vaginal Birth After Cesarean): A vaginal birth experienced by a person who has previously had a cesarean section delivery.

Cesarean Section (C-section): A surgical procedure in which a baby is delivered through an incision made in the abdomen and uterus of the birthing person.

TOLAC (Trial of Labor After Cesarean): An attempt to have a vaginal birth after a previous cesarean delivery. TOLAC is often recommended for individuals considering VBAC.

VBAxC (Vaginal Birth After x Cesareans): A vaginal birth attempted by a person who has previously undergone x cesarean section deliveries.

Scarred Uterus: A uterus that has previously undergone a cesarean section, resulting in scar tissue on the uterine wall.

Uterine Rupture: A rare but serious complication in which the uterine wall tears during labor, potentially leading to severe bleeding and harm to the baby and birthing person.

Informed Consent: The process by which healthcare providers provide information about the risks, benefits, and alternatives of a medical procedure, allowing the patient to make an informed decision.

Induction of Labor: The use of medical interventions, such as medications or artificial rupture of membranes, to initiate or speed up the process of labor.

Active Labor: The phase of childbirth characterized by regular and strong contractions, cervical dilation, and descent of the baby through the birth canal.

Dilation: The widening or opening of the cervix during labor to allow the baby to pass through the birth canal.

Effacement: The thinning and shortening of the cervix in preparation for childbirth, measured as a percentage (e.g., 50% effaced).

Cervical Ripening: The softening and thinning of the cervix in preparation for labor and childbirth, often induced using medications or mechanical methods.

Fetal Monitoring: The process of monitoring the baby's heart rate and uterine contractions during labor to assess fetal well-being and detect signs of distress.

Episiotomy: A surgical incision made in the perineum (the area between the vagina and anus) during childbirth to widen the vaginal opening and facilitate delivery.

Perineal Tear: A tear in the tissue of the perineum that may occur during childbirth, classified by degree (first-degree, second-degree, etc.) based on severity.

Postpartum Hemorrhage: Excessive bleeding that occurs after childbirth, often defined as blood loss of 500 mL or more within 24 hours of delivery.

Birth Plan: A written document outlining the preferences and wishes of the birthing person regarding labor, childbirth, and postpartum care, including preferences for pain management, interventions, and support.

Doula: A trained professional who provides physical, emotional, and informational support to birthing individuals and their families before, during, and after childbirth.

Midwife: A healthcare professional trained in providing prenatal, childbirth, and postpartum care to low-risk individuals, often emphasizing a holistic and patient-centered approach to maternity care.

Obstetrician: A medical doctor specializing in the management of pregnancy, childbirth, and postpartum care, including both low-risk and high-risk pregnancies.

This glossary provides an overview of common terms related to VBAC and childbirth. It's important to familiarize yourself with these terms to better understand discussions and decisions surrounding childbirth options and care.

By providing comprehensive information on VBAC, addressing the concerns and needs of fathers, and empowering them to actively participate in the VBAC journey, "Dad's Guide to VBAC" aims to support and educate fathers as they navigate the process of vaginal birth after cesarean.

www.ingramcontent.com/pod-product-compliance
Lightning Source LLC
Chambersburg PA
CBHW070810260726

48660CB00005B/1789